The Person with AIDS

A Personal and Professional Perspective

Edited by

William M. Marcil, MS, OTR

Occupational Therapy Consultant
William Marcil Associates
Virginia Beach, Virginia

Kent N. Tigges, MS, OTR, FAOTA, FHIH

Associate Professor of Occupational Therapy
University of Buffalo–State University of New York
Buffalo, New York

SLACK Incorporated, 6900 Grove Road, Thorofare, NJ 08086-9447

SLACK International Book Distributors

In Japan
  Igaku-Shoin, Ltd.
  Tokyo International P.O. Box 5063
  1-28-36 Hongo, Bunkyo-Ku
  Tokyo 113
  Japan

In Canada
  McGraw-Hill Ryerson Limited
  300 Water Street
  Whitby, Ontario
  L1N 9B6
  Canada

In all other regions throughout the world, SLACK professional reference books are available through offices and affiliates of McGraw-Hill, Inc. For the name and address of the office serving your area, please correspond to

  McGraw-Hill, Inc.
  Medical Publishing Group
  Attn: International Marketing Director
  1221 Avenue of the Americas —28th Floor
  New York, NY 10020
  (212)-512-3955 (phone)
  (212)-512-4717 (fax)

AIDS and the Hidden Epidemic of Grief: A Personal Experience, by James P. Bell, pages 25-32, ©1988 by *The American Journal of Hospice Care*. Used with permission.

Lyrics from *Tommy*, page 70, excerpted from Townshend, P. (1968). *We're Not Gonna Take It*. Fabulous Music, Ltd., Essex Music, Ltd., BMI.

Figures 11-5 through 11-7, page 114, from Tigges, K.N. and Marcil, W.M. (1988). *Terminal and Life-Threatening Illness: An Occupational Behavior Perspective*. Thorofare, NJ: SLACK, Incorporated.

Editorial Director: Cheryl D. Willoughby
Publisher: Harry C. Benson

Cover based on a design by Donald Watkins, William Marcil and Kent Tigges.

Printed in the United States of America

Library of Congress Catalog Card Number: 88-43550

ISBN: 1-55642-098-6

Published by: SLACK Incorporated
               6900 Grove Road
               Thorofare, NJ 08086-9447

Last digit is print number: 10 9 8 7 6 5 4 3 2

Dedicated to the Memory of
Rick Denton

CONTENTS

Ch. 1, 3 - 6, 13 + 14

Appendices

Throughout this book, care has been taken to avoid the need to use gender-specific pronouns. In cases where gender was not specified and a pronoun had to be chosen, however, the male gender pronoun was used.

Acknowledgments

The production of any book inevitably becomes, at one time or another, a task of immense proportion and often seems to require the effort of what amounts to a small army to pull things together. We would like to thank the following people for their assistance in the production of this text:

Jackie Rankin and Jayne King for their incredible patience and composure when continually bombarded with manuscripts for typing and last-minute revisions. Their word processing skills are *par excellence*.

Don Watkins, Ruth Schultz and Barbara Evans of the Educational Communications Center at the State University of New York at Buffalo for their artistic expertise, graphics, enthusiasm and support.

The dozens of employees and volunteers of the numerous national, state and local AIDS organizations who gave input, support and direction to our effort. Jim Ebner and Louis J. Moran for direction, Jean McKinley, Danny Marcil, and Don Vandeusen for proofreading, input, and support.

Randy Shilts, Linda Aldand and all of the contributors. Without their expertise, this book would never have become a reality.

All of our colleagues, students, friends and families for support and encouragement.

Yvonne and Carol for love, support, proofreading, feedback and especially for putting up with us, once again, throughout this effort.

Finally, to you, the reader, for caring enough to take the time to read this book and to grow.

WMM
KNT

About the Editors

William Matthew Marcil, MS, OTR

William Marcil is an Occupational Therapy Consultant in private practice and AIDS educator in Virginia Beach, Virginia.

Kent Nelson Tigges, MS, OTR, FAOTA, FHIH

Kent Tigges is Associate Professor of Occupational Therapy, University at Buffalo, State University of New York. Formerly Director of Occupational Therapy, Hospice Buffalo, Inc., Buffalo, New York.

Contributing Authors

James P. Bell, BA was formerly volunteer coordinator at the Hospice of San Francisco, San Francisco, California.

Arlene Binkowitz is the mother of a person with AIDS and an AIDS educator in Long Island, New York.

Arnaldo Gonzalez-Aviles, MD is an instructor of psychiatry at Cornell University Medical College, which is a clinical affiliate of New York Hospital, White Plains, New York.

A. Billy S. Jones, MSW, CADAC was formerly the Director of Minority Affairs, National AIDS Network. He is currently on staff at MACRO Systems, Inc. and is a member of the American Psychological Association AIDS Community Training Project, Washington, D.C.

Missy LeClaire is an AIDS educator and consultant in Washington, D.C. She is the widow and former primary caregiver of a person with AIDS.

Mauro A. Montoya Jr., Esq is Director of the HIV Legal Clinic at the District of Columbia School of Law in Washington, D.C.

Victoria P. Schindler, MA, OTR is the Director of Rehabilitation Services and Coordinator of the Patient AIDS Education Program at the Forensic Psychiatric Hospital, West Trenton, New Jersey. She is also an Adjunct Professor of Occupational Therapy at Dominican College of Blauvelt, Orangeburg, New York.

Mary Tasker, MSW is Director of Social Services, AIDS Resource Foundation for Children, Inc., Newark, New Jersey.

Foreword

When I wrote my first news story on what we now call The AIDS epidemic, there were just 330 cases of the then-obscure disease in the entire United States. With each successive article, I would pull out my thesaurus to find new synonyms for "baffling" and "mysterious," because those were the adjectives that so often were required for descriptions of the syndrome. No one knew then what caused the disease; how it was spread was a matter of theory, not definitive fact.

It's hard to believe that my first story was written in April 1982, so recently and yet an eon away from our experience of the malady today. Now cases are counted in the hundreds of thousands worldwide, not the hundreds. The epidemic has claimed lives as disparate as Miss Kitty and Rock Hudson, Liberace and Roy Cohn. Every few months, a new category of celebrity is added to the AIDS roster: a congressman and a football player, a network television anchor and a famous artist. Of course, the epidemic spreads lethally among the far less celebrated as well, tearing from us our friends and neighbors, our cousins and uncles, our daughters and sons.

For our generation, this little acronym has become integrated with the cultural genetics of our time, symbolizing all that is fearful and deadly, all we would wish to avoid.

Even as science gives us growing hope for a medical solution to this epidemic in the not-too-distant future, we still live with the legacy of those fearful and mysterious times that marked the early years of the epidemic. They arise from time to time in the new news stories about discrimination, ostracism and shame, all phenomena that seem bound up in this epidemic.

However, if AIDS has given us a Gordian knot of complicated social issues to untangle, it is only because it resonates with so many deeper social problems, including homophobia, racism, drug addiction and the disparity in the quality of health care among the different economic classes of our nation. All these problems have long existed, but the AIDS epidemic has provided a powerful new spotlight to cast on them.

This new spotlight demands we confront these problems with one quality: urgency. The politicians prefer to talk about the need for compassion and indeed it's admirable that America has largely arrived at the consensus that people should not be kicked around when they're sick or dying. But compassion is not enough.

Compassion will not direct the services that are badly needed in major urban areas to provide humane and cost-effective medical care to those infected with the human immunodeficiency virus. Compassion alone will not help the hundreds of thousands of drug-addicted Americans overcome their chemical dependency and remove themselves from a collision course with the human immunodeficiency virus (HIV). Compassion may ease suffering but it in itself will not save lives the way expedited AIDS education and prevention programs can. Only substantive programs, executed with the utmost urgency, can perform these tasks. In a sense, it's time to move beyond compassion and make urgency the watchword of social policy concerning the AIDS epidemic.

If the following pages in this worthy book scream one word, it indeed would be urgency. No reasonable person can read from chapter to chapter and not be seized by the awareness that we need to mobilize our society to take on the challenges of AIDS. Every story here—whether of intravenous drug users or of children, of gay men with AIDS or the suffering of their mothers—carries this demand as its subtext and they also carry one moral: How well do we do as a society in meeting the demand of urgency, that more than anything else will measure our degree of civilization.

Randy Shilts
Guerneville, Sonoma County, California

Preface

This text was originally conceived as a companion text to our first effort: *Terminal and Life Threatening Illness: An Occupational Behavior Perspective* (SLACK Inc., 1988), which was written primarily for occupational therapists. This, in fact, remains the case. However, as our original idea began to develop, we felt that we were being somewhat parochial in directing a book on this topic to such a small segment of the allied health professions. Therefore, we have compiled this book in a way that, we hope, others will benefit from its contents as well. Due to the fact that we, the authors, are occupational therapists, other professionals may detect a slight bias in our presentation of the material. We do not mean to imply that occupational therapy is more important than any other health profession, for we all have an important role to play in this public health problem, it merely reflects our area of expertise within the health-care industry.

This book is not presented as an academic exercise per se but rather as a social, personal and emotional perspective of some of the poignant issues of the people who have been touched by this disease called AIDS. We have presented this as a text, although not in the traditional sense, by combining the formal approach of teaching with the informal approach. One cannot appreciate the depth of AIDS by merely reading the ever-changing AIDS statistics or by sifting through the alphabet soup of AIDS-related infections and drugs. AIDS is much more complex than that; it has a human side, as well. It is our hope that this text will provide the reader with both sides.

We have chosen to present the material contained within by employing a general systems format. General systems thinking allows us to view complicated problems as a whole, while simultaneously permitting us to see how the various subsystems can ultimately effect the higher levels of systems and super systems and how the lower systems are, in turn, directed by the higher. General systems theory has been used as a base for many learning and practice models, including occupational behavior and the model of human occupation.

In *Terminal and Life Threatening Illness*, Sherman wrote that "anything written about AIDS (in 1988) is necessarily written on the wind." This is certainly true in regard to the medical and scientific advances that have been made in understanding and combatting the disease. Information about AIDS, as well as the ranks of the afflicted, grow daily and some of the statistics and "current knowledge" may very well be antiquated prior to press time. Be that as it may, the higher- level problems and implications of the person, family and community levels will remain essentially the same. To be sure, many of these problems have not been addressed properly, if at all. It is these levels that we feel the reader should be most concerned with. It is time that we looked beyond the symptoms of AIDS and the lifestyles of its unfortunates. Our attitude must change from one of, "what can I do to protect myself?" to one of "what can I do to help make things better?"

Throughout this text, we use the term AIDS in a generic sense, unless otherwise indicated, to include the full spectrum of HIV- related illnesses (HIV-positive, asymptomatic, persistent generalized lymphodenopathy (PGL), AIDS-related complex (ARC) and AIDS). We recognize, and we hope that the reader will also, that there are definite differences between these terms and diagnoses. However, we feel that the reader will find the going easier without have to wade through the quagmire of tandem terminology.

The reader may notice that we use the term "innocent victims" of AIDS in regard to children. This is not meant to imply that others who have the disease are "guilty" and have brought it on themselves, for certainly no one would willingly choose such a destiny. To be sure, all those afflicted by HIV are innocent victims. However, children are often viewed by society as innocent because they typically do not engage (willingly) in the high-risk behaviors associated with HIV transmission. It can be said that most, if not all pediatric AIDS cases are as the result of situations that are totally out of their control.

For those readers who desire to find specific information at a glance, we have included what we consider to be salient in the appendices and the glossary.

Finally, this book has been compiled by the efforts of both professionals involved in AIDS-related work and experts on AIDS. The professionals are those who have earned their degrees through the university system and are currently involved, either directly or indirectly, with the problem of AIDS. The experts—the only *true experts*—are those persons whose lives have been directly affected by AIDS; either as one who is in some stage of HIV disease and who knows, all too well, its manifold ramifications, or as a family member, friend or lover of someone who currently has AIDS or has died from the disease. In some cases, the experts and the professionals are one and the same.

This book does not attempt to answer all questions about the disease of AIDS. Quite frankly, we do not know them all—no one does. AIDS is too complex an issue. Neither is this a "how-to" book about AIDS. The primary objective of this work is to educate the reader about the complicated nature of this disease and, perhaps, to provide some insight into the needs of those who are affected by it. Education is the greatest tool we have at our disposal if we are to solve the conundrum of AIDS. It is our desire to replace the cold statistics of AIDS with faces—faces of people who have needs and desires just like everyone else. People who have a need to contribute to society in some small way, and who ask for nothing more than understanding and a chance.

William M. Marcil, MS, OTR
Kent N. Tigges, MS, OTR, FAOTA, FHIH
Buffalo, New York

AIDS Self-Knowledge Test

True—False—Unsure or I Don't Know (?)

T	F	?	1.	If a person tests positive for HIV, that means he/she has AIDS.
T	F	?	2.	If a pregnant woman has HIV or AIDS, her baby could be born with it.
T	F	?	3.	HIV is transmitted the same way that measles, mumps and the flu are transmitted.
T	F	?	4.	Donating blood can put you at risk for HIV.
T	F	?	5.	IV drug users transmit HIV to one another through the contaminated blood in needles and syringes they share.
T	F	?	6.	People with HIV or AIDS should not work in restaurants because they can transmit this condition to their customers.
T	F	?	7.	Using latex condoms when engaging in oral, vaginal and anal sex is the most effective way of preventing HIV infection and other STDs.
T	F	?	8.	Using a condom always prevents transmission of HIV.
T	F	?	9.	Kids with HIV or AIDS pose a risk to classmates when they attend school.
T	F	?	10.	Women who have sex with women are not at risk for becoming infected with HIV.
T	F	?	11.	Drug and alcohol use contribute to HIV transmission by impairing a person's ability to practice 'safer' behavior.
T	F	?	12.	HIV can infect the brain, causing mental problems.
T	F	?	13.	Once someone is infected with HIV, he/she will become ill and die within 3 months.
T	F	?	14.	People with AIDS look and feel perfectly healthy for long periods of time.
T	F	?	15.	Most people who have HIV don't know they have it.
T	F	?	16.	Women can give HIV to men.
T	F	?	17.	The symptoms of HIV infection vary greatly from person to person.
T	F	?	18.	Almost 1/4 of all U.S. AIDS cases are found in New York State.
T	F	?	19.	Most infants with HIV or AIDS get it from a blood transfusion.
T	F	?	20.	AIDS is a problem for public swimming pools, bathrooms and saunas.

Source: The American Red Cross of Western New York. Used with permission.

From: The Person with AIDS: A Personal and Professional Perspective, Marcil & Tigges.

PART ONE

The Personal Perspective

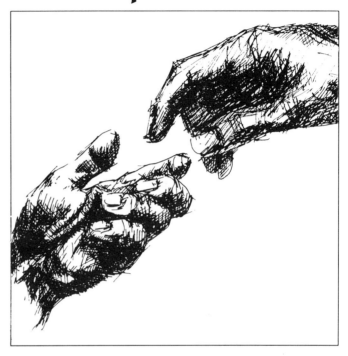

We must realize that we all have AIDS; Every man, woman and child; that we all have AIDS in our consciousness, and that we must work together as a human community against this disease.

—From the journal of Barry Binkowitz, MD

It is very important for people to realize that we are fighting a disease. We are not fighting a person or a lifestyle.

—Missy LeClaire

1 AIDS and the Human Dimension

William M. Marcil, MS, OTR

Lord, make me an instrument of Your peace.
Where there is hatred, let me sow love;
Where there is injury, pardon;
Where there is despair, hope;
Where there is darkness, light;
And where there is sadness, joy.
O Divine Master, grant that I may
seek not so much to be consoled
as to console;
to be understood as to understand;
and to be loved as to love.
For it is in giving that we receive,
it is in pardoning that we are pardoned,
and it is in dying that we are born into eternal life.
—The prayer of St. Francis of Assisi

Introduction

It is difficult to believe that it has been more than a decade since the first few cases of a mysterious and deadly disease began to trickle into hospitals and clinics in New York and California. That trickle soon became a steady stream of people; mostly gay men, for whom medical science could do little and whose cries for help went virtually unheard by the general public. It was almost two years after these first few cases that this disease was given a name: acquired immunodeficiency syndrome (AIDS), now the most feared acronym of the twentieth century.

In its relatively short lifetime, AIDS has killed over 100,000 American men, women, and children (CDC, 1991), and the toll rises daily. The statistics are staggering, especially if we consider that in the 11 years of the Vietnam conflict, 58,000 Americans died! On the other hand, however, if we consider that the Spanish flu epidemic of 1918-1919 killed over 500,000 Americans, or that automobile accidents and various forms of cancer, together claim over one million lives per year, the number of AIDS deaths somehow seems inconsequential in comparison. Why then, does this little four letter word frighten us so?

Issue I: Rejection and Isolation

Disease has always mystified and terrified people. There has always been a disease that impacted a given generation since the beginning of recorded history. One of the earliest examples is leprosy. Lepers were treated with disdain and ostracized from society; they were forced to live in isolated colonies, away from the mainstream. Today, the term "leprosy" remains synonymous with rejection and, interestingly enough, leper colonies, in one form or another, continue to exist throughout the world. In medieval Europe, the bubonic plague, also called the Black Death, caused the deaths of some 25,000,000 individuals. Its victims were treated with a similar lack of compassion and understanding. Special protective garments were often employed by physicians when treating its victims. Those who were fortunate enough to escape infection avoided those who were not so fortunate. The plague is another term that is frequently used to describe rejection. It is interesting that both leprosy and the plague have been used extensively as comparisons when people speak of AIDS in modern society.

There have been, and continue to be, other diseases that have vexed the human race: smallpox, syphilis, tuberculosis and polio, to name a few. Although these maladies have since been controlled through medical advances, the individuals who were stricken continued to be banished from the mainstream, into new "leper colonies": sanitoriums, rest homes, developmental centers, hospitals. The names have changed but the message remains clear: "We don't want you around us."

Along with the rejection and banishment, we seek to lay blame for a problem or disease on a convenient scapegoat. Leprosy, the Black Death, and even mental illness were long blamed on the Devil. An outbreak of food poisoning in colonial Massachusetts led to the infamous Salem witch trials and the execution of a number of innocent young people deemed to be witches. Syphilis, long a major cause of illness and death, was referred to by the British as the "French disease," while it was simultaneously deemed "the British disease" by the French. We have treated AIDS in the same manner. We blame the African green monkey, the African people, the Haitians, but mostly we blame the gay community. We term AIDS the "gay plague" or the "gay cancer." Many feel that the victims of AIDS deserve what they get and possess a certain amount of smug *schadenfreude*—the feeling of pleasure in others' pain. Laying blame may make us feel better, but it does nothing to solve the problem.

Issue II: Intolerance and Denial

As horrible as some diseases such as leprosy, multiple sclerosis and cancer may be, AIDS is particularly distasteful to many in the community. Aside from the often hideous nature of the disease process itself, and the Pandora's box of symptoms it produces, AIDS has forced us to deal with issues and problems that we have conveniently closeted away over the years: sexuality—specifically homosexuality—and intravenous drug use. We dislike having our closets opened and our skeletons rattled about.

Our society is basically intolerant of those who prefer to be intimate with members of their own sex. Many within our society view homosexuality as being "sick," "deviant," or "unnatural." Although the climate has changed somewhat since the sexual revolution of the 1960s and the gay liberation movement of the 1970s, the intolerance largely remains. Many states have laws that prohibit acts of "sodomy" between two consenting adults, even in the privacy of their own home. It is no longer socially appropriate to tell racial or ethnic jokes, but gay jokes are okay. Some people believe that it doesn't matter what gays think or feel. They don't count. They don't matter.

We dehumanize homosexuals. We forget, or actively choose not to consider, that they, too, are human beings. They are doctors, nurses, teachers, construction workers, actors and politicians. There are gays who are social deviants, just as there are heterosexuals who are. They have families and friends who care about them, and they contribute to society in a variety of ways. The only difference is that they express their affection in a way that is different from the norm.

Society's rejection and denial of homosexuality played a role in the slow progress in identifying and combatting AIDS. Because it was not a problem that affected the general population, interest in and funds for AIDS were generated at a snail's pace. It was only when the disease was seen as a threat to the heterosexual community that the money and interest began to grow. However, the denial continues. For example, in the New York State prison system, where there is an extremely high incidence of AIDS among inmates, condoms are not distributed because "homosexuality is not allowed" and therefore, condoms are not necessary. Similarly, many churches condemn both homosexuality and heterosexual sex outside of marriage on religious grounds. Because condoms are a form of birth control, their use is prohibited. People are getting mixed messages. Right or wrong, there will always be homosexuals and there will always be sex outside of marriage. A condom can save a life. As the denial continues, so will the spread of AIDS. This is not meant to imply that abstinence does not have a place in modern society, for it most certainly does. To be sure, abstinence from non-monogamous sexual relationships and from the use of intravenous drugs is the only sure way to prevent the spread of AIDS. Abstinence is a worthy option for many people. However, it is something that must be taught from a very early age and must be reinforced over time. This educational process is the job of the family and of the church. If these values are not instilled in every child as soon as they are old enough to understand, how can they be expected to overcome the temptations that are brought about by hormones and reinforced by peer pressure?

Issue III: The Innocents of AIDS

Our fear of AIDS and our anxiety engendered by homosexuals has been generalized to others who have fallen victim to this unfortunate disease. Those who have contracted HIV through blood transfusions, or through unknown means, are thrown into the same camp and receive the same unfair treatment by society. Ryan White, of Indiana, and the Ray brothers of Arcadia, Florida, all became HIV-infected through contaminated blood products used in the control of their hemophilia. Although many perceive infection in this manner to be "innocent," these individuals all received the same harsh treatment by their respective communities. Unable to attend school, unable to participate in their communities, shunned and despised, they were banished to their homes, which became their very own leper colonies. To add insult to injury, they were harassed, insulted and threatened by some in the community. All were jeered at and called "faggots." The Ray family endured the greatest harassment: their house was burned to the ground. All of this in America. All of this because of something over which they had no control.

There are thousands of "innocent" victims of AIDS; those who received their fate prenatally. Many of these children possess a dual diagnosis of drug addiction and HIV/AIDS before they have even begun to breathe. This has given rise to the increased number of "boarder babies" who live their short lives in hospitals and foster homes because their families cannot or will not care for them.

Issue IV: AIDS as a Tool for Racism

Since AIDS first came to our attention it has been regarded, by and large, as a disease that affects homosexual and bisexual men more than any other group. For this reason most AIDS funds have been directed at this group in terms of education and treatment. The gay community has mobilized and has become a formidable political force. Lobbyists and groups such as ACT UP have drawn political and public attention to their cause. The unfortunate consequence is that these groups appear to benefit primarily white, middle-class gays and, as a result, a large segment of society—a segment at extremely high risk for contracting AIDS—has been neglected. This group is comprised of nonwhite men, women and children who are primarily Black or Hispanic.

Taken together, Blacks and Hispanics comprise only 18 percent of the total population of the United States. However, these groups currently comprise almost 50 percent of the total number of AIDS cases. Certainly, these figures demonstrate a disproportionate ratio across our society. However, these statistics should not be surprising when one considers that minorities have always been held in small regard. Society has provided this group with inadequate resources in both education and health care. Despite the Emancipation Proclamation and the civil rights movement, we have kept minorities enslaved in a vicious cycle of ignorance, illiteracy, unemployment, poverty, crime and disease. As a society, we profess that "all men are created equal" yet we deny many the opportunity to rise above their lot in life. We keep minorities segregated into ghettos and housing projects, taunting them with the carrot and stick of equal opportunity while allowing very few to actually achieve it. It is no surprise that many turn to illegal means such as narcotics trafficking, larceny and prostitution to survive, let alone to achieve the "American dream." Of course, we as a society cannot tolerate these enterprises and we incarcerate the offenders—the ultimate in slavery. We then look at our prisons and see that Blacks and Hispanics comprise over 80 percent of the population—reinforcing our preconceived notions that these people will never make it within our society despite all of the "opportunities" that we have provided them with.

On the other hand, minorities have not readily undertaken the issue of AIDS as a threat to their well-being. They have dealt with it the same way that the majority has dealt with it—through denial. Although drug abuse has, arguably, become a fact of life in most inner cities, it is not a subject that many want to discuss—especially if it directly involves them or a loved one personally. Intravenous drug use is a subculture unto itself. Aside from being the most efficient means of transmitting diseases such as AIDS and hepatitis, it is a vehicle for spreading these diseases to a large and varied group of people, either directly by the sharing of needles among addicts, or indirectly through sexual contact between an infected user and a non-using partner which can ultimately lead to an infected child born as a result of these unions. AIDS has become another link in the shackles of segregation.

If homosexuality is difficult for the white middle class to accept, it is virtually impossible for those in Black and Hispanic communities to accept. Although there are many gays and bisexuals in this population, they tend to become less a part of their own subcultures and more a part of the gay subculture which, again, is predominantly white and middle class. This severe denial and rejection of homosexuality has been a major obstacle in the prevention of AIDS within the black and Hispanic communities. There is a great deal of trepidation on the part of national and community leaders to address the issue of AIDS or to seek help from AIDS organizations because AIDS is still viewed as a "gay disease."

Even in death, AIDS is denied. No mention is made of AIDS at the funeral of a 20 year-old man who was a known intravenous (IV) drug user, if a funeral is held at all. It is so much easier and socially acceptable to say that one died of cancer—an individual or his family cannot be blamed or stigmatized by cancer. Denial, therefore, allows AIDS to continue to proliferate within the community.

Are we using AIDS as a tool for racism and segregation, intentionally or not? Do we have a hidden agenda by keeping AIDS in the ghetto and denying the proper resources to prevent its further spread? Can the leaders of these minority communities overcome the specter of AIDS so that they may mobilize to overcome this new Sword of Damocles which sways tenuously over their heads?

Issue V: AIDS as a Disease of Society

We fear those things that we do not understand. We mask our fear with self-righteousness and hate. We forget that those afflicted with an unfortunate circumstance, a disability or a disease, are human beings. If it does not affect us personally, we want no part of it. Often, it is not until we ourselves are personally touched by a similar circumstance that we can see the other side of the story. AIDS is not something that anyone would elect to have. No one wants to live from day to day never knowing if it might be his last. No one wants to endure the pain and disfigurement caused by a pathologic invasion. No one wants to suffer the social pain of abandonment and ostracism. No one wants to give up everything they ever loved, including life itself.

AIDS is more than a disease that ravages the body; it is a disease that ravages our society, as well. AIDS does not affect merely a single person either. Although a given individual may be infected, that person's personal constellation is also dramatically affected by the disease. We are so focused on the diseased individual that we overlook the mothers, fathers, sisters, brothers, spouses and children who are involved. In our efforts to protect ourselves from the disease, we ignore the subtle impact on the various cultures and subcultures that comprise our communities.

AIDS affects all of us, at every level of our existence. The effects of the disease touch us at many levels—from the smallest of cells, to the basic unit of society, the family—to the levels of local, national and international policy. As Barry Binkowitz has written, "We all have AIDS" in one way or another, whether we want to admit it, or not.

We are a human community and, as such, we must all work together in the fight against AIDS. The fight is not just against the virus itself, but also against the fear and loathing of its victims—for we are all its victims. Each of us has an important role to play in this battle. Some of us may play a more important role than others, but we each have a mission—no matter how trivial or unimportant it may seem.

Not everyone is willing or able to work directly with people with AIDS, just as not everyone can work with other groups of people in need: the severely handicapped, burn patients, those with psychiatric disorders, or geriatric populations. Just because one cannot or will not work with one or more of these populations, does not make one a bad person. We all have our limitations and it is important that each of us recognize our own. What is important, however, is that we lend our support to others who may choose such work. We all need help and support in our daily lives; this is what makes people special. We must be tolerant and accepting of those with HIV disease, their families, their lovers and their caregivers. We cannot and must not be judgmental about how or why they contracted the disease; that is no longer the issue.

There is no doubt that science will eventually discover a cure or vaccine for AIDS. This remains to be seen. In the meantime, however, we must still deal with our present situation: the tens of thousands who are HIV infected and the hundreds of thousands, perhaps millions of people who are at risk for contracting the virus. AIDS may eventually fall by the wayside and be relegated to the status of other diseases such as tuberculosis and polio: controlled but not eradicated. However, we can be fairly certain that a new disease will eventually loom on the horizon; an "Andromeda Strain" that, perhaps, will be much more sinister, more unrelenting in its course, more easily transmitted, more deadly. Will we deal with such a disease in the same manner that we have dealt with AIDS? What lessons have we learned in the past decade?

2 The Psychosocial Issues of AIDS

Victoria A. Schindler, MA, OTR

Let me not pray to be sheltered from Dangers but to be fearless in facing them.

—Rabindranata Tagore, *Fruit Gathering*

Introduction

AIDS is an illness of loss. Like suicide or abortion, it has been described as an "unspeakable loss." Despite the fact that it is such a devastating illness, it remains a difficult subject to discuss. Because of this, it is more difficult to get solace, and mourning is more complex. This issue of loss affects not only the person with AIDS, but also the worried well, HIV-seropositive individual, persons with ARC (PWARC), and families, friends, lovers, and health-care workers of persons with AIDS.

The issues of loss may begin to surface as soon as the person realizes that he may be at risk for having contracted the virus and will continue in a variety of forms as long as the person is living with HIV. The issues may become more acute at times of crisis, and at times may appear to be resolved, but will never be forgotten.

All of the issues deal with loss and will affect every aspect of the person's life. However, the issues are also individualized and the depth of impact will vary from person to person. This chapter will first focus on the issues as they relate to the person affected by HIV, then address the issues of the families, friends, and lovers of the person affected by AIDS, and finally address the issue of health-care workers who work with people affected by AIDS.

Psychosocial Issues for Persons Affected by the Human Immunodeficiency Virus

People with whom I have worked who have been directly affected by HIV state that life has now taken on two dimensions: before AIDS (BA), and after AIDS (AA). The difference between the two began the moment that they first suspected they were HIV-positive, and they state that life has not been, nor will ever be the same again. Although most psychosocial issues have usually been addressed to the person with AIDS (PWA), it does appear that these issues start with the worried well, and if that person receives a positive result to an HIV antibody test, these issues continue in a variety of forms for as long as that person is living with HIV.

Worried Well

The worried well population consists of those persons who currently believe that their present or past behavior has put them at some risk of contracting HIV. This group includes persons with realistic concerns regarding their potential to contract the virus in addition to those who unrealistically perceive themselves to be at risk. On medical testing, the worried well person is asymptomatic of AIDS-related conditions. However, various psychological and physical illnesses may often be seen in this population as a result of their concern about their condition. The worried well may experience depression, anxiety, panic attacks, and a total preoccupation with the issue of AIDS. This concern can also manifest itself physically in the form of constant headaches, fatigue, gastric disturbances, and hypochondriacal AIDS-like symptoms such as weight loss and lethargy.[1,2]

Some members of this group may not have been tested for the virus as of yet or may have tested negative for the virus in the past but are now worried that their behavior since the negative test result may have put them at risk. Several other factors in addition to the person's high-risk behavior may also influence their concern regarding their potential to contract the virus. The person may live in a major metropolitan area in which AIDS is constantly in the news (e.g., New York or San Francisco) or may be a health-care worker who is constantly reminded of the threat of AIDS.[1,2]

One of the major psychosocial tasks for the worried well individual is to make the decision as to whether to be tested for the virus. While people are at this stage of decision making, they may be acutely anxious and may be consulting family, friends, health-care workers and others to obtain information to make a decision. Consulting with sources who can give accurate, objective information may help to alleviate some anxiety associated with the antibody test, while frantically searching for answers may only serve to further instigate misconceptions. Others may feel so overwhelmed by the prospect of being HIV-positive, that they may not be able to verbalize any of their feelings or questions about the virus and may avoid the issue, or turn to the media for information. This, too, may serve to further disrupt their lives.

While worried well individuals vacillate in the decision-making process, they may experience a variety of feelings associated with the process itself. The feeling of ambivalence about whether to be tested or not often leaves one very unsettled and uncomfortable. Guilt is also often experienced. Persons may worry about whether they have infected others since they have not yet sought an answer regarding their own condition. They may also feel guilty about causing undue worry to significant others if they have consulted them about being tested, or may feel guilty about a "secret" they are holding from others if they have not yet shared their concern about the virus or their high-risk behaviors.

Several factors have been identified as benefits and risks of HIV testing. Some of the benefits are that it may encourage those with high-risk behaviors to reduce or eliminate those behaviors and adapt a lifestyle with an increased emphasis on proper nutrition and health care and safer sex. It can help women to decide whether to pursue or avoid pregnancy, and can be used to support a medical diagnosis for an unexplained illness. Also, it can greatly alleviate anxiety about whether one has been exposed to the virus or not, especially if the result of the test is negative. On the other hand, testing also carries risks. Many choose not to be tested because they prefer to feel anxious about their condition, rather than deal with the absolute knowledge that they are HIV-positive. Also, the knowledge that one is HIV-positive can lead to a host of feelings that will be discussed further in the next section.[3]

Now that knowledge has been increasing about the issue of AIDS, worried well individuals can utilize hotlines and anonymous testing sites that offer pre- and post-test counseling. These resources, in addition to other medical and social resources, can provide concerned persons with current, accurate, and objective information regarding the HIV virus and antibody testing.

The HIV-Positive Asymptomatic Person

Persons with HIV may require a great deal of adjustment on receiving the positive result of their antibody test. Although estimates on the likelihood of developing AIDS among HIV-infected individuals vary from 20 to 78 percent,[4,5] once a person learns that he is positive for the HIV virus, it is quite normal to react initially with feelings of fear and doom. HIV-positive individuals are suddenly faced with the issue of contagion and must worry about transmitting the virus to others, protecting themselves from opportunistic diseases, and dealing with the responses and fears of lovers, family members, friends, coworkers and the public. The first few months following a positive test result leave the person vulnerable to reactive psychiatric symptoms of depression, anxiety, and preoccupation with the illness. This vulnerability to AIDS-related distress may continue to affect the person at various times throughout the course of the illness and appears to be tied into the various unknowns about the illness.[6]

Especially for those individuals with a history of poor coping skills and limited social supports, the danger of an intense psychiatric reaction is possible. Some persons may experience suicidal thoughts. Therefore, families, friends, lovers and health-care workers should stay attuned to changes in psychosocial functioning so that professional help can be sought in a timely manner. Although many individuals have responded with suicidal gestures on notification of their results, the majority are able to handle this information with the proper supports and resources. HIV-positive individuals need to be reminded that they are in a psychosocial crisis as opposed to a medical crisis and should seek out support to cope with this information.[2,3]

Once the initial reaction begins to subside, the individual needs to deal with issues regarding changes in his lifestyle. Studies are now showing that individuals who do go on to develop AIDS or ARC may live with the positive HIV result for seven years before developing any symptoms.[7] However, throughout this time the person must acknowledge that they are infected with the virus and can transmit it to others. Therefore, sexual practice, IV drug use and pregnancy are major issues for this population.

It is imperative that the individual understand the modes of sexual transmission and adhere to safer sex practices. Individuals may overreact to this and eliminate all intimate behavior including non-modes of transmission such as hugging. Especially because sex is a major mode of transmission, persons may develop much difficulty in their sexual relationships despite knowledge about safe sex practices. Guilt, unrealistic fear, and avoidance of developing an attachment to another person can get in the way of developing a healthy sexual relationship. This is unfortunate, since most HIV-positive individuals are young adults who would otherwise find sexuality to be a prominent issue at this point in their lives.

Other individuals may avoid safe sex practices. For some, the use of condoms is often a negative issue. Studies have documented that there are several barriers to using condoms. Some see condoms as unnatural[8,9], ineffective[10,11], offensive to the partner[12,13,14] and an embarrassment to purchase.[15,16] Other negative thoughts on condoms are that they reduce spontaneity in sex and can reduce the pleasure of intercourse.[1,7,17] Some persons, out of anger, have knowingly infected others.[18] If a person can be assisted to seek out information regarding safer sex, resources such as self-help groups and AIDS hotlines can assist a person in obtaining appropriate safer sex information.

Intravenous Drug Use

Intravenous drug users (IVDUs) are the fastest growing population of seropositive individuals. The rate of HIV infection among IVDUs in the New York metropolitan area is currently 50-60 percent and recent information states that it is not unreasonable to believe that one of every two IVDUs in substance abuse treatment is already infected with the HIV virus.[4] Most cases of heterosexual transmission involve IV drug use, and, therefore, the growing number of pediatric cases are tied to an IV drug user or a partner of an IV drug user.[3] Because of this dual mode of transmission with this population, education must be directed toward the risks in sexual transmission and needle sharing behaviors.

Recent studies are beginning to show that IVDUs are responding to some of the warnings regarding AIDS. One long-term residential substance abuse treatment center reported that the knowledge of an HIV-positive result enhanced, rather than undermined, the effectiveness of treatment.[4] However, other reports describe that IVDUs are less likely to modify their sexual behavior.[3]

Society disapproves of IV drug use, and this further compounds the difficulty that the IVDU faces on a positive test result. The person may already be alienated because of antisocial behavior, ostracized by family and friends, have difficulty functioning at work, or be unemployed and have marginal daily living habits such as poor nutrition and sleeping patterns. This, in addition to a positive HIV result, can lead to further rejection and alienation. In addition, IVDUs, as opposed to gay men, do not have an organized community to rally for their needs. Therefore, IVDUs will usually face a variety of psychological reactions upon confirmation of a positive result in addition to a strong sense of having "wasted their life"—especially the parts of their life that have been focused on IV drug use.[3,4]

Because most cases of heterosexual transmission involve IV drug use, the majority of pediatric cases are emerging from relationships in which one or both parents are IVDUs. In most cases it is the man who is the IVDU, and who has transmitted the virus to the mother of the child.[3] In addition, the women who run the highest risk of infection are those who are most socially and economically disadvantaged and delay seeking treatment.[1] Unfortunately, many of these women are of childbearing age.

Current estimates now state that a child has a 50 percent chance of testing positive for HIV when born to an infected mother. Because of this, women need to know that the virus can be passed on to the fetus during pregnancy and to the child via breast feeding. This limit on the childbearing process can be highly depressing and stressful. Women will need to grieve for the children they dreamed of but are now unable to have.[1]

Persons with AIDS-Related Complex

The major psychosocial issue for the person with ARC is the fear and anxiety regarding whether or not their illness will progress to a life-threatening form of ARC or if it will progress to AIDS. Because of this, a diagnosis of ARC is often seen as the "beginning of the end" or a sign of impending doom. Although the definition for AIDS has been revised with the 1987 Centers for Disease Control (CDC) case definition[19], and now includes symptoms and illnesses that were previously defined as ARC, a diagnosis of ARC is still a devastating event for the person. In fact, the diagnosis of adjustment disorder was more often made in persons with ARC than persons with AIDS.[6] In a comparative study of gay men with AIDS (N = 89), ARC (N = 39), and no physical symptoms (N = 149), ARC patients scored at least as high, if not higher, than AIDS patients, on multiple parameters of both general and AIDS-specific distress. This is believed to be secondary to the persistent uncertainty about developing AIDS.[6]

Once diagnosed with ARC, the person must begin to face the persistent nature of multiple medical problems. This may involve hospitalizations and periods of absence from work and other daily activities. Questions about financial entitlement, ongoing employment, insurance and legal issues may become topics that now need to be dealt with rather than just questioned. The person may now begin to take on the sick role and all of the issues of dependency and helplessness that accompany it. If the person is already involved in support groups, this may indicate a move from a seropositive group to a PWARC group. This combination of physical and psychosocial stress may require additional support.

Persons with AIDS

The actual diagnosis of AIDS had been shown to be an extremely critical period that can often be filled with mixed reactions. For some, the diagnosis of AIDS may come after years of knowing of one's seropositivity and dealing with ARC conditions. For others, it may be a complete surprise, accompanied by an intense reaction. This particular group of PWAs may need to face issues of homosexuality and drug abuse—often for the first time.

Paradoxically, some have found the diagnosis to be a relief in that they no longer need to worry if they will develop AIDS or not. Whatever the case, the PWA is immediately faced with issues of loss and the threat of impending death.[2,20,21]

The issues regarding loss and death are profound and affect every area of life. However, the issues affect each person differently and what may be a devastating loss for one person may be a minor loss for another. Also, what may be a devastating loss for a person at one given period of time, may, at a later period of time, be resolved, lose some of its importance, or may resurface and become an even stronger sense of loss. The impact of loss depends on each's individual goals, values, and priorities, and on the lifestyle the person had prior to their learning of the AIDS diagnosis.

These losses can also be defined in terms of their effect on the normal life activities for the person affected by AIDS. Because the virus usually strikes persons in young to mid-adulthood (25 to 45 years), it has a huge impact on the life cycle tasks of this period. To understand the impact of the individual types of losses, they will first be described in their relation to the overall impact on the life cycle and then will each be described individually.

Overall, at this point in the life cycle, the adult is expected to enter new roles of responsibility at work, home, and in society, and develop the values, attitudes, and interests attributed to these roles.[23,24]

Work usually becomes a major focus and the young adult is expected to choose an occupation that will provide a livelihood for himself and possible dependents. Much time and energy is spent on this process, and work becomes a central part of the adult self-concept. Leisure is now viewed as a time of earned recreation and relaxation from work and often takes the form of exercise, sports, and hobbies.[23,24]

Socially, young adults are in a period in which they usually will become less dependent on their parents and, instead, form an intense commitment to another person or a cause, or become withdrawn, lonely or self-centered. Sexuality is a powerful drive and there is a need to find adequate and satisfying sexual experiences. Physiologically, the young adult has reached his optimum mental and motor functioning. Thinking and learning are objective, realistic and problem-centered, and the body is usually at its peak of functioning. In fact, this is the point in which many athletes reach their highest level of performance.[23,24]

PWAs are suddenly thrown to a much later developmental period without adequate opportunity to master the life tasks for young adulthood. This new time period now includes persons who are 20 to 40 years older and encompasses tasks of retirement from work, separation or loss of intimate relationships, and decreased physiologic and mental functioning.[23]

These new tasks of retirement and social, physiologic and cognitive loss are difficult for those who are naturally going through them, since they are associated with the aging process and impending death. They are rarely seen as joyful, anticipated life experiences, like the tasks of marriage or job establishment. To master this period of the life cycle, people need to accept the aging process and death, perceive their life as useful and productive, and engage in activities that are compatible with their actual physical and psychological capabilities. This is quite difficult to achieve at 65 years of age; the expectation that a person will be able to conquer these tasks at age 35, when productivity has recently begun, and death is still supposedly 30-40 years away, can be inconceivable.[23]

However, now that PWAs are living for several years after they have been diagnosed with AIDS, they need to face these drastic changes in life tasks.[23,25] These changes are directly related to the issues of loss that are associated with AIDS, and the tasks and the issues combined give a sense of the overwhelming effect of this illness on a person's life.

A loss that encompasses many areas is a loss of life roles. These life roles may include the role of worker, student, friend, lover, or family member. Additionally, due to the questions about AIDS and the inability of a PWA to predict the future, many PWAs experience difficulty in setting or maintaining career, personal and social goals.[22,23]

Due to financial, medical or other reasons, the PWA may no longer be able to work. This incapacity not only results in financial problems but often in a loss of identity if work had been an important part of that person's life. Often the person may have spent months or years in school or training for a much-wanted career only to now be faced with a very premature retirement. Also, since many PWAs may be too sick to work, yet too well to stay home on a consistent basis, they may be left with much unstructured time, which results in a feeling of decreased productivity. If the person happens to be a student who is embarking on a career or attempting to further their career with additional training or college, these goals have to be greatly modified or put on hold on a temporary or permanent basis. These changing career goals, especially after they had been planned over long periods of time, can be extremely disappointing.

Persons affected by AIDS also experience a loss of social roles. Fatigue and medical restrictions and changes in cognitive, physical and psychological functioning can cause the person to limit social participation. Leisure, the time that had been reserved for refreshment from work, may now become the major focus of the person's schedule, and some recreational sport activities may no longer be viable due to the person's decreased physical status.[3,22] Additionally, the person may be experiencing the loss of some of his social supports to AIDS-related illnesses and to death. In addition to the person having limited capabilities to reach out to others, the persistent yet unwarranted fear of contagion can cause previous social contacts to withdraw their support. Due to feelings of helplessness or a fear of mortality, family and friends may withdraw their support. Although sexuality is usually powerful at this stage, the person with AIDS may experience a weakened sexual drive, decreased sexual capabilities, loss of sexual partners, or may experience guilt or conflicting feelings regarding sexual practice, since it is a method of transmission of the disease. This sexual repression can lead to aggression or an increase in alcohol and drug use. All of this can result in a PWA viewing himself as a leper in a social and sexual void.[3,6,22,23]

The loss of roles is directly related to massive lifestyle changes and an alteration in the quality of life. Not only may the person experience decreased financial earnings, but also the financial cost of treatment may be overwhelming. Daily habits and routines may be disrupted and may be replaced by frequent hospital appointments and exorbitant amounts of time devoted to issues of third party reimbursement or government financial aid.

All of these roles and changes can be further affected by the dementia process. Recent information is showing that AIDS-related dementia is having a profound effect on AIDS patients and may often be the first sign of AIDS. This dementia is a direct infiltration of HIV to the brain and can drastically change cognitive processes and personality moods. This may start subtly; with early changes noted in forgetfulness, decreased motor abilities and social withdrawal, and can progress to global disorientation, paralysis and mutism in their terminal stage. Because of this overwhelming nature of dementia, it alone can severely alter one's functioning in all of the life tasks.[26,27]

These massive changes evoke varying but strong psychological reactions which have often been depicted as an "emotional rollercoaster"[2] of responses. Although a variety of reactions will be described, their level of priority or profoundness varies for each PWA since this can only be described by each individual experiencing the loss at that time.

Denial

Denial has been described as an unconscious means of resolving conflict and relieving anxiety by disavowing thoughts, feelings, wishes, or needs, which are consciously intolerable.[28] For persons faced with a life-threatening illness, denial can be a useful defense mechanism, since it can give them some control over how they will handle the issue of their own mortality. Denial can promote optimism and allow the person to continue functioning and be as productive as possible. This can be somewhat more difficult for PWAs since they are constantly faced, via the media, with the reality of their illness and the high mortality rate associated with it. However, denial should be fostered, and PWAs should be encouraged to avoid dealing with death on a daily basis. This method is usually accepted by most PWAs since they really are people who want to live and do not want to be consumed with dying.[22]

Fear

Fear is another intense reaction experienced by PWAs and has a wide scope. One of the greatest fears is fear of social abandonment. Due to unwarranted issues of contagion, many PWAs fear they will be abandoned by family, friends, lovers and other significant people. This abandonment can begin with the loss of work colleagues and acquaintances and progress throughout a person's support system. In addition to fears of contagion, other issues regarding sexual orientation or drug use may further alienate the PWA from family and friends and lead to abandonment. Lovers may realistically fear they have been exposed to the virus, or may themselves be ill and unable to care for the PWA. In addition, the PWA may have already lost friends or a lover to AIDS which would further reduce their social support and cause more fear regarding the loss of supports which are available. This can all be compounded by the ultimate form of abandonment-rejection by society.

PWAs also fear a loss of self. This can include a fear regarding loss of roles, in addition to disfigurement and a loss of body functions. With all of the present information on the incapacitating and disfiguring effects of some of the neurologic disorders, the mental deterioration, and the wasting syndrome, horrifying pictures of the later-stage AIDS patient have developed. This picture of oneself as marred and deformed is terribly frightening. Unfortunately, this fear is only compounded with the fear of pain which accompanies all of these maladies. In fact, PWAs have stated that they fear the pain and disfigurement associated with AIDS more than death itself.[22,29]

PWAs also rightfully experience a fear of the unknown. Although much information has developed about AIDS, there is still much that needs to be discovered. This lack of answers can cause fear regarding new tests or procedures to issues regarding one's length of time to live. All this fear can lead to tremendous anxiety.

Sadness

With all of the changes in life roles and bodily functions, the PWA can experience intense feelings of sadness and depression. This may surface for short periods of time, especially at times of crisis, or may present as a constant, dull, aching feeling. The sadness may be accompanied by crying, isolation, anhedonia, or feelings of suicide. Some PWAs may be able to request and receive individualized means of support at these times, while others may continue to deteriorate psychologically, and may require professional psychiatric assistance. At this point the PWA may be diagnosed with an adjustment disorder or a major depressive disorder and placed on therapeutic medication. As mentioned previously, although some PWAs do commit suicide, the majority are able to seek assistance to remedy these intense feelings of sadness.[20,22,30]

Guilt

Guilt is another feeling that is often experienced regarding the issues of AIDS. PWAs may experience guilt regarding past behaviors that led to infection or regarding the fact that they may have unknowingly infected others. In cases where a PWA may have knowingly infected others, he may later feel guilt for this behavior. For those who continue to view their homosexual orientation or their inability to control their IV drug use as immoral behavior, they may view AIDS as a punishment. For gay men, this can emerge as "internalized homophobia" which is an adoption of society's prejudicial attitudes. Behavior is then viewed as deviant to society and is accompanied by feelings of guilt for not obeying social mores. This guilt can be crippling and result in a decrease of productive energy to fight the battle of AIDS.[22]

Anger and Rage

Anger and rage is another response to all of the losses and issues associated with AIDS and is a reflection of the injustices of a terminal illness and a rejection by members of society. These feelings can be channeled productively into issues such as fighting for the cause of AIDS or by being assertive with one's doctor or family regarding one's needs and wishes. This anger and rage can also be used unproductively in acting out behaviors such as physical destruction of oneself or others, or knowingly infecting another individual with the virus. Support systems can help an individual to identify this anger as appropriate and to channel and release it in productive ways.

The effect that the alteration in life roles and psychological reactions will have on the PWA, or anyone infected with the virus, is now being linked to the type of personality the individual has had prior to AIDS and the coping skills and resources available to the person to deal with this type of medical and psychosocial crisis. If a person is able to view their infection with the virus as a realistic result of bad luck, or of behaviors that were unknowingly linked to the virus at the time they were performed, the person has a much better chance of dealing with AIDS in a more productive way. On the other hand, if the person views their infection with the virus as a result of being a bad, immoral person or as an act of revenge for some action, they are less likely to cope in a productive manner. Persons who have had extraordinary high goals and standards, and rigid, inflexible routines will also have more difficulty adapting to the constant fluctuations and unknowns accompanied by AIDS. Persons who have a history of pre-morbid psychological dysfunction, such as a person with a psychiatric disorder or long-term IV drug use, will most probably experience more intense difficulty due to their already limited psychosocial functioning and coping skills. For this group, sexual acting out and drug use may have been means of coping with stress in the past.[22]

Information has recently become available on the linkage between pre-morbid personality, coping skills and survival rate for PWAs. Long-term survivors have been found to maintain good relationships with others, maintain intimacy to death, and ask for, and receive, medical and emotional support. Additionally, although they do not focus on death as near, they do take it seriously and use their anger around this issue to draw others to them rather than to alienate them.[31] It has also been found that long-term survivors have been followed closely by their physicians and have had treatment initiated at the earliest signs of deterioration. The families of these survivors have had a strong commitment to the person's care and to providing the person with the necessary nutrition and health needs.[32]

On the contrary, short-term survivors have been found to have poor, destructive relationships, and to act in a manner that is viewed as passive, submissive, and fatalistic. These persons have less communication with health care staff and often lose interest in their condition.[31,32]

All of this information raises the question as to whether the length of survival is related to the mildness or severity of medical infections and/or due to a mind/body attitude that is closely tied to positive thinking, good health and nutrition, and social support. Some of the information gained in this latter area has come under the field of psychoneuroimmunology. This area of research relates stress associated immune suppression with AIDS and states that severe forms of stress have a direct relationship on decreased cellular immunity. It also describes that changes in immunity have their greatest impact on persons with already compromised immune systems.[33] To alleviate this stress, any resources that will serve to buffer or moderate a person's stress level, such as social supports, are viewed as helpful.

As described by Patrick Haney[29], a PWA, some positive things have developed from this extremely negative experience. AIDS has encouraged him to get in touch with his strength, live one day at a time, and to reconnect with his family and friends. AIDS has also allowed him to assert more power and control over his life through education and seeking treatment. Involvement in research projects, and AIDS volunteer organizations, can also assist one to feel more active in coping with AIDS. Although it can be extremely difficult to identify anything positive in this devastating illness, the attempt to do so does seem to appear to improve the quality and perhaps the quantity of life for the person with AIDS.

Families, Friends and Lovers

Families, friends, and lovers, and any other significant persons of the person affected by AIDS also develop psychosocial issues and crises and are in need of supportive care. Some of the issues experienced by each group overlap while other ones may be quite different.

At the same time that the family learns that their child or sibling is infected with the virus or has been diagnosed with ARC or AIDS, they may also be learning that the family member is gay or has a history of IV drug use. In a study conducted on the psychological repercussions of AIDS on family members, the most frequently cited sources of stress included: fear of contracting the virus, simultaneous revelations of homosexual or bisexual activity, in addition to the diagnosis of AIDS, helplessness associated with a terminal illness and social rejection. The study also found that communication between the PWA and the family was easiest among siblings and most difficult among PWAs and their fathers.[34] All of these stresses can be traumatic for the family and result in a variety of feelings.

For parents, the loss of a child can be devastating since it is perceived as being out of the natural order of life events. Siblings, due to the closeness in age and in at least some lifestyle habits, may develop fears regarding their own mortality. Family members, especially parents, may develop feelings of guilt or anger on discovering their child's difference in sexual orientation, IV drug use, or their child's sexual relationship with someone in one of the two categories, and may respond with shock or disbelief. Additionally, the issue of contagion may cause family members to isolate themselves from the patient. Despite the current evidence that the HIV virus cannot be transmitted in a casual manner, such as kissing, hugging, or sharing household items, family members who are not educated regarding this information or refuse to believe it, may continue to alienate themselves from the person with AIDS.[35,36] This unwarranted fear of contagion can spread beyond immediate family members. Extended family, friends, and significant others of the family of the PWA may alienate themselves from both the PWA and his family; especially if the PWA and the family reside in the same household. This can cause immediate family members to also experience a sense of social rejection from others.[21]

In some cases, family members may already be distanced from the PWA. In one study of 42 gay men, 62 percent reported having minimal or no contact with their family of origin. In some of these cases, issues such as IV drug use or homosexuality may be known at some level but may have been avoided by the family and the person with AIDS. These issues, or other family issues, may have created long-standing problems between the PWA and the family which neither party is willing to discuss or resolve. In these cases, the knowledge of the person's AIDS diagnosis may only serve to further distance the PWA from his family. Even if family relationships are adequate, the PWA may be significantly distanced geographically from the family. In fact, the above study also showed that 73 percent of the gay PWAs reported living alone and half of these relied on neighbors and friends, instead of families, for assistance. In some cases, a family member or several members may move to the PWAs home to provide care or the PWA may move to a family member's home. However, often this geographical separation does not allow for consistent communication between the PWA and the family.[22] In instances where the family of the PWA are involved and interested, there are support groups and educational programs available to meet their needs.

With many PWAs, lovers and spouses may be the most significant persons in their lives. These groups of people would have more of a realistic fear of contracting the virus. If the lover or spouse is already HIV-positive, he may require as much support as the PWA and the couple may have very little energy to mutually meet each other's needs. If the lover or spouse is HIV-negative, there may be a real fear of contracting the virus and this can compromise the sexual relationship. Issues of guilt and blame can surface, and these along with safe sex practices, need to be discussed in order for the sexual relationship to be able to continue in a satisfying way. If the PWA is too ill to be able to participate in sexual relations, the lover or spouse may need to find an appropriate way to deal with their sexual feelings.[21]

The lover or spouse will also experience feelings of intense sadness, helplessness, anger, and fear that would accompany the loss of a loved one to a terminal illness. In many instances, this person may experience these feelings more intensely than anyone else in the PWA's life. Therefore, the lover or spouse will need his own support system. If there is a good relationship between the PWA and the family, the family may also serve as a mutual means of support for the lover or spouse. However, in many cases, families have difficulty in viewing the depth of significance a lover has had in their family member's life. Therefore, support groups and educational meetings are also excellent means of support for lovers and spouses.

The significance of friends in a PWAs life may also be underestimated. Many PWAs may experience more commonalities and closeness with their friends than with their family and may have grown more dependent on their friends as their means of support. Therefore, friends can also suffer the same feelings related to loss as the family and lover or spouse and may also require supportive care. The same support groups and programs available to families, lovers, and spouses are also available to friends.

Whether the family, friends, and lover or spouse were with the PWA during a long, grueling illness or if they just learned of the PWA's illness at the time of death, the death itself is still a crisis for this group. It is important that all of the significant others are able to experience the grieving process. Certain rituals, such as funerals, memorial services, and participation in the Names Project Quilt[37] can assist with this process. Even after the death, bereavement support groups are available for significant others of PWAs.[30]

References

1. Cochran, S. and Mays, V. (1989). Women and AIDS-related concerns. *American Psychologist*, 44(3): 529-535.

2. O'Dowd, M. (1988). Psychosocial issues in HIV infection. *AIDS*, 2(Suppl. 1): S201-S205.

3. Christ, G., Siegel, K., and Moynihan, R. (1988). Psychosocial issues: Prevention and treatment. In V. DeVita, S. Hellman and S. Rosenberg (Eds.), *AIDS: Etiology, Diagnosis, Treatment, and Prevention* 2nd ed. Philadelphia: J.B. Lippincott, pp. 321-337.

4. Galea, R., Lewis, B., and Baker, L. (1988). Voluntary testing for HIV antibodies among clients in long-term substance abuse treatment. *Social Work*, May-June, 265-268.

5. Delaney, M. (Feb. 28, 1989). Staying alive: Making the ultimate political statement. *The Advocate*, 33-37.

6. Tross, S. (1987). Psychological response to AIDS and HIV disease. In J.C. Holland (ed.), *Current Concepts in Psychology and AIDS*. New York: Syllabus of the Post Graduate Course at Memorial Sloan Kettering Cancer Center, September 17-19.

7. Bolle, J. (1988). Supporting the deliverers of care: Strategies to support nurses and prevent burnout. *Nursing Clinics of North America*, 23(4): 843-851.

8. Darrow, W. (1974). Attitudes toward condom use and the acceptance of venereal disease prophylactics. In M. Redord, G. Duncan, and D. Prager (Eds.), *The Condom: Increasing Utilization in the United States*. San Francisco: San Francisco Press, pp. 173-185.

9. Felman, Y. and Santora, F. (1981). The use of condoms by VD clinic patients: A survey. *Cutis*, 27:330.

10. Hart, G. (1983). Role of preventive methods in the control of venereal disease. *Clinics in Obstetrics and Gynecology*, 18:243.

11. Armonker, R. (1980). What teens know about the facts of life. *Journal of School Health*, 50:527.

12. Arnold, C. (1972). The sexual behavior of inner city adolescent condom users. *Journal of Sexual Research*, 8:298.

13. Curjel, R. (1964). An analysis of the human reasons underlying the failure to use a condom in 723 cases of venereal disease. *Journal of the Royal Navy Medical Service*, 50:203.

14. Wittkower, E. and Cowan, J. (1944). Some psychological aspects of promiscuity. *Psychosomatic Medicine*, 6:287.

15. Yarber, Y. (1977). Teenage girls and venereal disease prophylaxis. *British Journal of Venereal Disease*, 53:135.

16. Yarber, W. and Williams, C. (1975) Venereal disease prevention and a selected group of college students. *Journal of the American Venereal Disease Association*, 2:17.

17. Condoms. (1979). *Consumer Reports*, 44:583.

18. Shilts, R. (1987). *And the Band Played On*. New York: St. Martin's Press.

19. Centers for Disease Control. (1987). "Update" HIV infections in health-care workers exposed to blood of infected patients. *Morbidity and Mortality Weekly Report*, 36(25):285-289.

20. Getzel, G. (1987). *Overview of the psychosocial issues concerning AIDS*. New York: Gay Men's Health Crisis Publications.

21. Christ, G., Wiener, L., and Moynihan, R. (1986). Psychosocial issues in AIDS. *Psychiatric Annals*, 16(3):173-179.

22. Christ, G. and Winere, L. (1985). Psychosocial issues in AIDS. In V. DeVita, Jr., S. Hellman and S. Rosenberg (Eds.), *AIDS: Etiology, Diagnosis, Treatment and Prevention*. Philadelphia: J.B. Lippincott, pp. 275-297.

23. Schindler, V. (1988). Psychosocial occupational therapy intervention with AIDS patients. *The American Journal of Occupational Therapy*, 42(8):507-512.

24. Murray, R. and Zentner, J. (1979). *Nursing Assessment and Health Promotion Through the Life Span*, 2nd ed. Englewood Cliffs, NJ: Prentice-Hall.

25. Guiles, G. and Allen, M. (1987). AIDS, ARC, and the occupational therapist. *The British Journal of Occupational Therapy*, 50(4):120-122.

26. Buckingham, S. and Van Gorp, W. (1988). Essential knowledge about AIDS dementia. *Social Work*, March-April:112-115.

27. Price, R. and Brew, B. (1988). The AIDS dementia complex. *Journal of Infectious Disease*, 158(5):1079-1083.

28. American Psychiatric Association. (1980). *A psychiatry glossary*. Boston: Little, Brown.

29. Haney, P. (1988). Providing empowerment to the person with AIDS. *Social Work*, May-June:251-253.

30. Govoni, L. (1988). Psychosocial issues of AIDS in the nursing care of homosexual men and their significant others. *Nursing Clinics of North America*, 23(4):749-765.

31. Greenfield, S. (1989). The health care team-partners in caring. Conference Presentation at New York University, New York, February 10.

32. Holtz, H., Dobro, J., Palinkas, R., et al. (1986). Psychosocial impact of the acquired immune deficiency syndrome (letter to the editor). In H. Cole and G. Lundberg (Eds.), *Journal of the American Medical Association—AIDS from the Beginning*. Chicago: American Medical Association, p. 117.

33. Glaser, R., and Glaser, J. (1988). Stress associated immune suppression and AIDS. In T.P. Bridge, A.F. Mirsky and F.K. Goodwin, et al. (Eds.) *Psychological, Neuropsychiatric and Substance Abuse Aspects of AIDS*. New York: Raven Press, pp. 203-215.

34. Frierson, R., Lippman, S., and Johnson, J. (1987). AIDS: Psychological stresses on the family. *Psychosomatics*, 28(2):65-68.

35. Friedland, G., Saltzman, B., Rogers, M., et al. Lack of transmission of HTLV-III/LAV infection to household contacts of patients with AIDS or ARC with oral candidiasis. *The New England Journal of Medicine*, 314(6):344-349.

36. Friedland, G. and Klein, R. (1987). Real and perceived risks of AIDS in the family and household. In *AIDS: Information of AIDS for the Practicing Physician*, Vol. 3. Chicago: American Medical Association, pp. 16-22.

37. Boodman, S. (1987). Giant quilt names 1,920 AIDS victims: Memorial will be unfurled on Mall (Washington DC AIDS Rally. *Washington Post*, 12 October, p. 110.

3 AIDS and the Hidden Epidemic of Grief

A Personal Experience

James P. Bell, BA

Will all our lives become a faded memory that is lost in time when we have just begun to understand the meaning of our lives?
Danny Marcil, *As Dreams Go By*

AIDS has become the most feared disease of this century. Since 1981, 100,000 people have died in the United States from this disease, with new cases being diagnosed daily. At present there is no cure in sight. The financial strain on the health-care system is growing. AIDS patients in San Francisco spend an average of 40 days in hospitals at an average cost of $1,000 per day. As the number of cases increase, hospital beds become increasingly scarce, and limited resources are spread thin. State and federal governments are committed to provide more funding for research, treatment, and education, yet volunteer organizations carry much of the burden.

The hidden epidemic of AIDS is an epidemic of grief. For every AIDS patient that dies there are at least five bereaved—parents, whose children have died; friends, who have lost countless friends; lovers, who are now alone. As the deaths from AIDS mount, the hidden epidemic of grief spreads quietly among the population. What follows is one person's story of personal losses due to AIDS. It is not written from a clinical viewpoint. It is the personal experience of one of many who have lost someone to AIDS. The writer has lost 87 friends, which is not uncommon in a city where some have lost up to 200 friends and others have simply lost count. This large number of losses means that many have lost their entire social network and support system. The grief experienced is not only for the loss of friends, but also grief for the loss of a way of life and the concurrent attitude adjustments necessary for survival in the midst of an epidemic. This, then, is my story of grief, loss, and survival.

The story actually begins in April 1975, six years before the beginning of the AIDS epidemic. That was the year I was honorably discharged from the Army.

Separation pay and discharge papers in hand, I came to San Francisco to start a new life. For three months I spent time learning about the city. Eventually I went to work for a large corporation, bought a car, and moved into a house which I shared with a friend. It was a year of hope and new beginnings. The future was bright with endless opportunities. It was the year I came to terms with my sexuality, and I spent the next three years reveling in the sexual freedom found in San Francisco.

Those three years were full of activity. I had a full-time job and was moving up rapidly in the corporate world. Within a year I had gone from the mailroom to entry-level management. It felt good to be successful. At the same time, I attended a university at night, carrying a full course load. I managed to complete my degree with a respectable grade point average. I remained in the Army Reserve, partly to maintain access to PX and commissary privileges. I worked as a psychiatric technician one weekend a month and two weeks a year for additional training. My social life did not suffer one iota, as I was out almost every night, and spent my free weekends going on short trips. I was so busy having a good time and being successful that I had neither the time nor the desire for a serious commitment to another person; besides, there were "so many men, so little time." However, I did establish a social network of friends and acquaintances. I also had countless sexual encounters.

Eventually I grew weary of the fast life. The pace was too fast—I felt like I was not savoring life's moments, but gulping them down in great swallows. The quality of my relationships was not good. I had surrounded myself with a crowd of good-time-Charlies who had no interest in the serious side of life. There were a few exceptions, but my social group consisted mostly of frivolous people lacking motivation to pursue interests other than sex, drugs, and alcohol.

Thus, in 1979 I became involved with the Hospice of San Francisco as a patient care volunteer. Motivation to volunteer for anything is never purely altruistic, and I was no exception. While my primary motive was to serve those in need, I had a multitude of other reasons for volunteering. One goal was to meet a higher calibre of people than I had met in bars, baths, and discos. I chose hospice work because I had not experienced the death of anyone close to me, and I felt a need to work with death and loss so I would be able to handle the deaths of my loved ones when the time came. Two years later I had fulfilled my personal goal of learning about death and grief, and I had established a higher quality of social life. My desire to serve remained strong and grew stronger as other goals were met. What I had not anticipated were other changes, specifically a new list of priorities for my own life. One of my goals was particularly strong, and needed to be fulfilled at an early age. I had always wanted to live outside the United States and experience the life of an immigrant, to see the United States from the outside and to experience living in another culture. In early 1982 I moved to Canada, a country not far from home and where English is a primary language.

As I was preparing for the move, I began hearing rumors about a few gay men with strange illnesses, but they were a few isolated cases, and no one I knew had heard anything more. I gave it no more thought and set out for Canada.

For the next two and a half years I heard little about AIDS, or anything else from the United States for that matter. While I lived only 30 miles from the U.S.

border, news from the States was sketchy and dealt mainly with economics and politics. There were no publicized cases of AIDS in Canada at that time. AIDS was an American disease, and was "not too infectious." This was the extent of my knowledge of AIDS. It was something that happened to other people in other countries. Letters from friends were not any more enlightening, but I found it odd that friends stopped writing, one by one, until I received no letters at all from San Francisco. The cliche "out of sight, out of mind" seemed relevant, so I assumed friends had stopped writing because I was no longer a part of their lives. My life was so busy in Canada—hospice volunteer, member of the board of directors of the local crises center, full-time job, and a small business of my own. There was no time to dwell on matters far away in another country that had no effect on my life.

The life of an immigrant was not easy—the prejudice in Canada against foreigners was subtle but strong. Because of that, the poor economy, and the constant dreary weather, my decision to return to San Francisco was an easy one. By June 1984 I was ready. I was excited, anticipating reunions with old friends, revisiting familiar haunts, and getting back to life at home. I called a friend, told him of my plans, and asked to stay with him for a few weeks until I could get settled. He agreed, but warned me to prepare myself for the changes that had occurred over the past three years. When I pressed him for an explanation, he refused to elaborate, simply warning me to prepare for a shock. He said we would talk when I arrived in San Francisco. I hung up, and with a sense of foreboding wondered, "just how serious is this AIDS thing?"

It was the middle of July 1984, and the weather was hot. I packed my car and drove straight to San Francisco, stopping only for gas. It was a long, hot drive and I was exhausted when I arrived in San Francisco at 1 a.m. I stayed in a motel that night rather than disturb my friend. It was good to be back home, and I fell asleep anticipating reunions with old friends. I slept well. When I arose the following morning, I called my friend and drove to his apartment. We had a short visit, with much discussion of my trip back. I unpacked a few things while he dressed for work. We talked about his school, family, the summer Olympics in Los Angeles, everything but AIDS. He was anxious to get to work, and I to tour the city. I gave little thought to what we did not talk about, assuming we would discuss AIDS later. I dropped him off at his office, and immediately went to check out my old hangouts on Castro Street, formerly THE place in San Francisco for a gay man to go. The image in my mind—a hot, July afternoon and crowds of people on the street—could not have been further from the reality that greeted me as I approached the Castro. The street was empty.

Three years earlier the sidewalks teemed with crowds of smiling faces; now, there was no one. The bars and stores, once filled with shoppers and daytime revelers, stood empty. Several businesses had closed down, gone bankrupt, or simply moved away. I also noticed that of the few people on the street, many were women. What had been the gay male enclave was now a mixture of gay men, lesbians, and heterosexual men and women. I perceived this as a positive change. It seemed the polarization between gay men and lesbians and heterosexuals was much less than three years earlier.

I went back to my car and headed off to another predominantly gay area,

Folsom Street. Three years earlier there were at least 20 gay establishments along the street, stretching for at least a mile, thus earning the street the nickname "miracle mile." Now, driving down the street, I saw only seven, four of which would close in the next year. These changes made it seem as though I was in another city, in another time. Others had several years to see the gradual changes and adapt. I saw them in a matter of hours and had to readjust immediately. I attributed the changes to the AIDS epidemic—hundreds had died, thousands had either moved away or were spending less time going out and more time at home. The full horror of the epidemic would hit later.

I headed back to my friend's apartment, a cloud of fear hanging over my head as I thought of calling my former friends. I got back to the apartment and began going down my list of phone numbers. I made the first call and heard the recording, "The number you have dialed has been disconnected, and there is no new number." Sixty calls, 60 recordings. My heart sank and fear and panic set in. Where were all my friends? The people I ate with, lived with, worked with, and played with; where did they all go? I sat there, numb and confused, denying the possibility that they were dead.

My friend returned from work, and I told him about my day and the phone calls I had made. He pulled out of his footlocker copies of obituaries he had been saving for the past three years. This was his way of remembering the dead. In those yellowed columns were the names of 57 of the friends I had tried to contact. Only three friends were left, and one of those had moved to Mexico. My heart was ripped out and torn apart.

He told me what it had been like as the epidemic spread—first trying to name the disease, going from GRIDS to AIDS, the stories of bus drivers refusing to stop in gay areas, beatings, deaths, the ultimate association of sex with death, righteousness of fundamentalist religious groups, apathy of government, fear. There were many stories, stories of fear, sometimes of terror, always of horror. This is what I had returned to—a plague city. He explained safe sex, a term and concept new to me, and he explained sexual behaviors that were considered safe. I learned about AIDS, the various opportunistic infections associated with it, symptoms that may indicate it, and I also learned that there was no cure.

I heard about how San Francisco was beginning to respond, a response due in part to pressure from the gay community. I heard about volunteer groups founded to provide care where no one else would. I heard about persons with AIDS, rejected by family, church, government, and society, being cared for by members of the gay community, many of whom would themselves succumb to AIDS. The epidemic was, and still is, horrible. In the midst of this horror, the best of human nature appeared. For each horror story of rejection there were ten stories of compassion and care. If there was no hope for a cure, there was hope in people and hope that compassion would conquer fear.

The next several weeks were a blur. It took that long for the shock to wear off and to realize the enormity of the task I was about to undertake. I had expected a relatively smooth transition. Instead, I was faced with adapting to some changes on a very basic level—readjusting to American culture and a new code of sexual behavior, establishing new friendships and a completely new social network, finding a job and apartment, and grieving my losses. If I wanted to survive, I had to adapt fast. Some things needed to be done immediately, and some things could be delayed. I thought my grief could be put off, so I buried it deep inside, and kept it there for far too long.

In the span of a month, I had found the job, the apartment, and made the other necessary adjustments. But I did not look at my grief. I began to make new friends. Slowly my life began to move forward. One step in that forward motion was to return to the Hospice of San Francisco as a volunteer. In October 1984 I returned as a patient care volunteer with the newly formed AIDS Homecare and Hospice Program of Hospice of San Francisco. This was to lead to my first face-to-face contact with AIDS.

I met my first patient in his hospital room, and as I had in the past with other patients, developed a rapport with him. Sometimes volunteers can identify closely with the patient, both the same age, similar education, similar backgrounds. This can cause difficulties for volunteers, because the volunteers see themselves on the deathbed and become overwhelmed with fear and anxiety.

I had worked with young cancer patients in the past, so over-identification was not an immediate problem. However, I was taken aback by the unusual and unnecessary precautions used by some staff at the hospital, such as wearing masks, gloves, and surgical gowns when merely entering the room. I was surprised because the Hospice of San Francisco rarely recommends this procedure for casual visits. Eventually my patient, who had also become my friend, died and I was assigned to another. I saw more people with AIDS, and in their wasted faces I could see the faces of the 57 of my friends who had died. These were my peers, members of my community; they were dying and there was nothing I could do. I felt helpless. My grief began to surface, but I was too afraid to face it, so I buried it deeper.

In February 1985 I joined the hospice staff as the volunteer coordinator for the AIDS program. This position allowed me to see the full list of names of the hospice caseload all at one time, instead of one patient at a time. At first it was painful watching my peers die one by one, some of whom were friends, others nameless sexual encounters from years past. Soon my own fears began to surface—when will I get it? Am I next? Is this cold more than a cold? What's that spot on my leg? Eventually I became resigned to living in the midst of the epidemic; each death was like a brick piled on a brick piled on another brick. So this is what grief felt like—not depressed, not sad, just weighted down. I quickly buried the pain of my new grief with the rest. I saw new friends become sick and die—another brick. I saw volunteers become sick and die—another brick. In the midst of an epidemic, as in war, some people die, some people live, and for the survivors the load of grief gets heavier, some carrying more pain than others, but most also burdened with the question, "Why not me?"

My closest and oldest friend returned from Mexico in 1986. He was concerned about a sore on his foot, "from stepping on a piece of glass at the beach." I recognized it as Kaposi's sarcoma (KS), the cancer associated with AIDS. Because I am not a doctor, I did not share my opinion with him, but suggested he see his doctor and have his foot examined. He went for a biopsy, which tested positive for KS. He suffered for 10 months and died in January 1987. That was it—the last brick.

All my losses caught up with me. My grief could no longer be held in abeyance. The pain and the grief swept over me—it was the beginning of my dark night of the soul. His death cut the last thread to the past; I no longer had any old friends. The pain of my grief hit hard. It was as though I was floating in darkness, on a sea of pain, blown by the winds of rage. There was no hope, no light. I pulled into myself, cutting myself off from the world to protect myself from more pain. It hurt so bad all I wanted to do was to cry. I became furious at God and threw Him out of my life. The Great Comforter, source of consolation, lifted not one finger to help, even as I begged for relief. He had deserted me, left me on my own to fend for myself. I became sharp and caustic to everyone, pushing all away. Going to work, to the death house, was repugnant. It took every bit of strength to get up in the morning. I lost my appetite—food tasted like dust in my mouth. I could not sleep at night, nor stay awake by day. Dazed by the force of my grief, I wandered through each day. I wanted to scream and cry until I had no screams, no tears, left. But I didn't. I stayed lost in ever-present pain, ate with pain, worked with pain, went to bed with pain. It was my constant and unwelcome companion. I would wake up in the middle of the night, gasping for breath, unable to breathe, being choked by pain.

I desperately needed to get away from all responsibilities for a time, to be by myself, and to let go of the pain. I hated work, and when I took a week off in March 1987, I did not want to return to my job. This shocked me, as this was the type of job I had wanted all my life. On a deeper level, I knew that quitting was not the answer. It was at this point that I realized I was grieving all my losses, and I could not delay dealing with my grief any longer. I was burning out because of my grief.

I was at the point of burnout, not wanting to quit my job, but not wanting to go on either, and unable to think clearly enough to decide either way. It was time for my annual evaluation, and it was the opportunity to talk with my supervisor about what was going on with me. I summoned up all my nerve and told her how I felt. The ensuing discussion we had was very good. My supervisor provided me with a third option—a leave of absence. While the job evaluation was not the best, it was fair. My supervisor was supportive and empathetic. She saw I needed time to grieve, and gave me the month of April 1987 off. Her support helped me accept my grief, which was the first step in working it out. As I left the office on the last day before my leave, I wondered if I would return, and honestly at that point I didn't care.

The first weekend passed quietly. The following Monday was a different story. I slept late, and when I finally did get out of bed, the house was quiet. The hard knot of pain that had settled in my heart began to loosen and move up, up my chest to my head, and out through tears and wailing.

The next two weeks I cried until there were no more tears. I screamed until my throat was raw. I sulked in silence. I began to relive all the memories of my friends, laughing about the good times, crying about their deaths, allowing my anger because I felt cheated out of saying goodbye to them. I wrote letters to each one, saying the things I had not said in the past, things I had wanted to say. I wrote a goodbye to each, and then burned them all. As the smoke rose into the sky, I let my pain rise with it and let it go. The third week I rested, exhausted.

With the pain gone, I began to see clearly. I included meditation as part of my daily routine. The darkness was lifting and light began to enter my soul. Interest in life reawakened within me. I started noticing the small details of everyday life, the change of season from winter to spring, the return of some birds, the trees putting out new leaves. My perspective became more balanced. I discovered that the God I accused of deserting me had been there all along, and had answered my prayers, not by taking the pain away, but by letting me experience and work through the pain. By this time 80 of my friends had died from AIDS, and the losses were indeed painful. But as I have experienced many losses, I could see my many gains and the good things in my life: a significant other who cares very much about me and who was with me through this dark time, never complaining or criticizing, always patiently listening and accepting. Without him, I would have had a much more difficult time. I have new friends who are as wonderful as the ones who are gone. I have fulfilling job, which allows me to be creative and gives me a good deal of freedom and responsibility. I work with warm, caring, supportive people. Finally, I have my health and life. All these will one day pass, as one day I will also die. Now is the time to cherish what I have.

I returned to work and began to see the world in a different light. I began to feel more open, more sensitive to the needs of those around me, more tolerant of human weakness in others and in myself. I have time and energy to hear what others are saying and to allow them their feelings. When someone experiences a loss, I am slower with the words, for I know what is more important is an accepting presence.

A month was only the beginning, but it allowed me to release the pain I had buried for so long. I think back to those who are dead, and I am sad. I have a long way to go in my grieving process, but at last the tremendous burden of pain is gone, and I am beginning to feel whole.

The burnout I experienced is gone. It was not the job that led to burnout, but rather the manner in which I dealt with my grief. During that month of leave, I traced the pattern that had led to burnout. First, I isolated myself and withdrew from any support that was available. Next I denied the pain, thinking falsely that I had to be strong for others. I became confused and lost clarity. What I have learned is another way to deal with my grief: share it with people close to me in my support system, and resist the temptation to pull into myself; be open to myself and listen to what my heart is telling me, no matter how painful. Meditation helps me maintain clarity and to keep everything in perspective. I take each situation one at a time, rather than jumbling everything all up into one big mess.

There is a myth that to reach burnout is to be a failure, and to admit burnout is a recognition of failure, and that once burned-out there is no turning back. It is not failure to be overwhelmed by tremendous losses, but, for survival, it is necessary to realize when I need time to take a break.

There are many other changes that have begun—my attitude, perspective, methods, of dealing with problems, and how I see myself and others. I'm becoming less judgmental, more tolerant of human weakness in myself and in others. I recognize my faults more readily and am becoming more patient. I feel more freedom in my life. These changes are still new, and I have to work hard to incorporate them into my daily life. Old habits and ways of thinking don't die easily. I still make many mistakes and will continue to make mistakes, and I don't always do as well as I could. I know that I am at the beginning of a long journey and still have much work to do. But, I have learned to be the victim of circumstances, and I have a choice in how to respond to life's ups and downs. I have learned to be patient with myself during this journey, and not to rush my grief. Through the suffering and pain, I have gained the strength and the tools to survive in this epidemic and to continue to be of service to those in need.

We are all affected by AIDS and the mounting deaths. I reached a saturation point in my personal and professional life where I could not fit in another death. The cumulative deaths have an effect. Those caring for persons with AIDS need to take time off at some point to release the grief and sorrow and to reconnect with life and living things. To admit that one needs time away is not an admission of failure, but a request to survive, to continue on in this work, and to be available to the growing number of persons with AIDS and the bereaved.

4 Living with AIDS
A Woman's Point of View

Missy LeClaire

In my time I have been called many things: sister, lover, priestess, wisewoman, queen. Now in truth I have come to be wise-woman, and a time may come when these things need to be known.
—Morgaine in Marion Zimmer Bradley's
The Mists of Avalon

I cannot remember what my life was like before AIDS. AIDS was certainly not a class that I would have signed up for-but it has taught me much about life, people, and most of all, myself. In just a few short years my life, like the lives of thousands of others, has been changed forever by this disease. I have realized that there is no "after AIDS"; once it touches you, it stays with you always. I have discovered too, that I have the stamina, the will, and the wherewithal to be a long-term survivor.

Jim and I met in Ocean City, Maryland, in early 1985. He was a merchant marine who spent two weeks of each month at sea. As I was extremely independent, this was a wonderful way to develop a relationship—I had time with him and time to myself, too. At six feet, three inches and 185 pounds, tall, dark, and handsome, Jim was the picture of health. He was a man who worked hard, played hard and loved life. We had a 10-month torrid romance and were married in December of 1985. Around that time, Jim began to show an obvious weight loss. We assumed that the weight loss was due to the stress of relinquishing his bachelorhood, accepting new employment, and relocating to New Jersey.

During February of 1986, Jim had a work-related physical. Even though he complained to the doctor, an occupational specialist, of the recent weight loss and growing fatigue, the doctor told him that he was in tip-top shape. In April of 1986, Jim called me on ship-to-shore radio and asked me to make a dental appointment for him. He told me that he had a serious "gum infection" and that he was concerned. I assured him that I would do so immediately. Remembering his recent weight loss and fatigue, I also decided to make a doctor's appointment, as well. Because I had no AIDS knowledge at this time, I certainly didn't know any of the signs or symptoms of the disease.

By the time Jim arrived home, he was so fatigued he could hardly walk, and his throat was so sore, he could hardly swallow food. I found a general practitioner in our rural area to examine him; he stated that he had never seen anything quite like the symptoms that Jim exhibited. He sent us to an internist at the local hospital immediately. After numerous tests were performed, one of which was a non-consensual HIV test that was positive, no diagnosis was rendered. At one time, it was thought that perhaps the water aboard the ship was responsible for causing Jim's medical problems. One doctor said to Jim and me that, "It may be cancer or Hodgkin's disease; we don't know." We were left in the dark. I had purchased a book on AIDS at a local supermarket and, with the exception of the skin lesions, Jim had every AIDS symptom listed in the book. Jim now weighed 145 pounds.

Around this time, Jim developed urethral strictures as a result of a 1982 car accident. At that time, he suffered a broken pelvis and a severed urethra. He received eight units of blood after the accident. In June of 1986, Jim was hospitalized to relieve the strictures. This was to be our first encounter with the ignorance and stigma associated with HIV (or human T-lymphotropic virus, isolate III {HTLV-III}, as it was known at the time).

On the door of his isolation room was a sign clearly indicating that this patient was HIV-infected. His trays of food were left outside his door every day, and if I was not there each day, Jim probably would not have eaten at all. I did not see any staff members touch Jim. It was as if he had the plague. His medications were placed on his bedside table, and he was informed that they were there. His clean linens were left, folded, next to his bed. When I was unable to be there, he was left to fend for himself, alone in his hospital room. It was extremely disheartening to Jim and me. We had been through 10 weeks of uncertainty already and, for the first time, we fully realized that the ignorance of the AIDS virus existed in the hospital. Until that time, I thought that you entered a hospital to get well—not to be punished for your illness. Jim was swiftly released after surgery; although too weak to walk, he was sent home to recuperate with a catheter in place.

During this time, I had heard of a wonderful AIDS program at Johns Hopkins University Hospital in Baltimore, Maryland. I spoke with Dr. Newman who, after listening to my tearful account, asked me to bring Jim to Johns Hopkins as soon as possible. I was ecstatic, and discussed the situation with Jim's primary physician and the specialists we were working with. They were equally delighted.

The day before the appointment at Hopkins, I received an emergency call from Jim while I was at work. He was hemorrhaging. I rushed him to the hospital, where they applied a tourniquet to his penis and told me that once they "patched him up" I could take him home. I was gravely concerned and afraid to take him home for fear that the bleeding would begin again. Jim was already so weak, I was positive he would not be able to take any further blood loss. I called Dr. Newman who advised me to leave him in the hospital for that night. "If necessary," she said, "just walk out; they cannot put him out on the street." When I told the doctor (one of the specialists) that I was leaving Jim at the hospital, he turned on me in anger. "Don't you know that he probably has AIDS? I want him out of this hospital!" "That's too bad," I screamed back, "He's yours for the night!" I stormed out of the hospital. The next morning, I loaded Jim and his blood-filled catheter into the back seat of our car and began the 4-hour journey to Baltimore.

The acceptance we found at Johns Hopkins University Hospital proved to be the antithesis of our previous experience. The staff was warm and caring and were there because they *wanted* to work with people with AIDS. Jim was at Hopkins for three weeks. It was here that Jim received his official diagnosis of AIDS. He dealt with it the way many people deal with difficulties—he denied it. Two weeks after receiving his AIDS diagnosis he said to me, "No one has told me why we are here, we should go home." I replied that, yes, the doctors *had* told him, but, together with the program director, he was told again. This time he responded by withdrawing, both physically and psychologically, by pulling the covers over his head. He stayed like that, speaking to no one and eating nothing, for days. It was not until his father visited, from upstate New York, that Jim rejoined the world.

My family was very supportive, both financially and emotionally, during our crisis, and I will always love them for their care. They live in Washington, D.C., and have a small guest house on their property, which they rent out. When their tenant relocated to another area, they offered it to us, free of charge. We returned to New Jersey to pack. Jim was still feeling quite ill and exhausted and was unable to do too much during those hot July days. I arranged to sell our furniture and some stocks I owned to try to build up our empty bank account. Jim, being a "country boy," was not thrilled at the prospect of living smack dab in the middle of Capitol Hill, Washington, D.C., but he eventually adjusted. It was, after all, closer to Johns Hopkins and, more importantly, to a lifeline of different support systems.

To me, Jim was not the "typical" AIDS patient. He never developed pneumocystis pneumonia (PCP) or KS; his symptoms were more psychiatric than physical. During the first six months of his illness, he was severely depressed, angry, agitated, and almost manic at times. In fact, a nurse once remarked to me that working with Jim was very difficult. I responded, "If you were 27 years old and could not do a damn thing that you wanted to do in your life, how would you feel?" Yes, he was difficult and demanding, horribly so. Many critically ill AIDS patients are. People, especially health-care professionals, should realize that, here is an individual who, not only knows that he may soon die, but that he may most likely lose everything that he ever loved before death. Jim could no longer work, he was financially devastated, he no longer had much of a sex drive, he had lost contact with most of his friends, and he worried about the pain he was causing me and our families. His dream of the house with the white picket fence and three kids in the yard was shattered. Demanding? Angry? He had every right to be so.

When Jim wasn't in an agitated state, he would try to be his ever-loving, helpful self. He would have dinner ready when I came home from work; he would do laundry and handyman projects around the house. As the fatigue grew more taxing, and confusion set in, he went from Mr. Helpful to Mr. Do-Nothing. When I arrived home from work in the evenings, I would find him sitting in the same spot as I had left him in the morning, eyes staring straight ahead. The depression became so severe that he was confined to a psychiatric hospital for a few weeks.

Throughout November and December of 1986, however, he felt really well. He gained 35 pounds and was starting to look like his former healthy self again. By Christmas, however, Jim started to regress. The fatigue was back with a vengeance, along with a constant nosebleed. The weight started to fall off again. Eventually, he started to lose his short-term memory, as well. He would often ask, "What's for dinner?" a half-hour after a full meal. One vivid recollection I have is turning to see him standing by the bed in his socks, briefs and shirt, looking very confused. "What's wrong, honey?" I asked. Jim answered, "I don't know if I'm supposed to get into bed or get dressed." We had just returned from a vigorous 4-hour trip downtown to the doctor's office that he could not recall at all. At that moment, I remember thinking, "I'm losing my husband and my best friend, too!"

By mid-February of 1987, Jim was hardly able to get out of bed. He was becoming more and more confused and, at times, delusional. His anger, however, had all but disappeared. Because the Washington area had been besieged by two blizzards in as many weeks, I was unable to drive him to Baltimore to admit him to Johns Hopkins. His psychiatrist, the wonderful Jeff Ackman, MD, who practiced at George Washington University (GW) in Washington, D.C., suggested that Jim be admitted there. At that time, Jim finally received a diagnosis of dementia. Although I suspected that the dementia had begun long before, organic dementia was not considered to be one of Jim's problems. In fact, an earlier psychiatrist told me that Jim's strange behavior was due to an unresolved conflict that he had with his mother and had nothing to do with AIDS.

At GW, Jim was also diagnosed with *Mycobacterium avium intracellulare* (MAI) and told that he only had six months to live. Jim asked to spend his remaining time at home. MAI is a horrible multiple systems bacterial infection that ravages the body and causing extended fevers with temperatures as high as 106 degrees. I did not know that human beings could survive such high fevers; as usual, no one had warned or informed me of the frequencies and extremes of the fevers. Despite these high temperatures, Jim was unable to stay warm. The room temperature was kept at 96 degrees; yet, he shivered so violently that his body would literally lift off of the bed, regardless of the number of blankets I put over him, or how much of my own body heat I could give him. The MAI also caused some internal bleeding which, among other things, caused chronic nosebleeds that led to horrible sores. His Candida became uncontrollable. He lost 100 pounds between Christmas and his death in April of 1987. I think the most difficult thing for me to deal with was that, even though I was glad to be there for Jim and help him on his path to death, there was little I could do to alleviate his suffering. To watch him waste away and not be able to do anything about the situation was the most frustrating feeling I have ever had.

Towards the end, Jim needed constant care. I left my job to be with him 24 hours a day, seven days a week. It was exhausting, but I did it. He wanted to be home and I wanted him to be there. I contacted the local hospice for help, but they felt that we didn't need much skilled nursing care or health aide visits because I was "so efficient."

In contrast to my own, Jim's family was not a very close-knit one. His three sisters lived in Florida. His parents were divorced and each had remarried. They were, however, very supportive, even though the support was by long distance. Although AIDS did not drive his family apart, as it has so many other families, neither did it bring his parents any closer together. Each family member would make their own visits to see Jim. The girls would take their turns joining their mother and they were a tremendous help to me. They would come for a week or two and take over the cleaning, cooking, shopping, etc., providing a much-needed break for me.

The strain of being a caregiver was beginning to wear on me. I was made aware of, and began to attend, a support group for family members and significant others of AIDS patients. I allowed myself one night off each week to attend these meetings. Within the group I found others, mostly gay men, who were experiencing my same problems. The group provided my first insight into gay relationships; these men were suffering the same losses that I was and their commitment to their lovers was just as strong as my commitment to Jim. I found love, kindness, and strength within this group. It was a therapeutic aid to "recharge my batteries" for another week of crises. I found out the hard way that AIDS is not a disease that you can battle alone. You cannot handle this yourself as either a patient or a caregiver. You *must* have outside support. I'm thankful and grateful to my group for their responses to my critical situation.

Fortunately, in his last few months, Jim became less angry and less difficult to work with. It was as if he had finally reached an acceptance of his fate, and he was thankful for all of the love and support he received. He helped to make his own funeral arrangements and was adamant that they be carried out according to his wishes. He did not fear death, but frequently wondered what it would be like: How would he die? Would it be painful? Would he know death was approaching? Would I be there with him? Would there really be a white light? The doctors would never discuss the subject of death. I didn't know how to handle these conversations. We decided that, for him, dying would be like boarding a huge clipper ship and sailing out to sea on a beautiful sunny day. He seemed pleased with the notion of one last ocean voyage. After being semiconscious for two days, Jim died in my arms on the morning of April 22, 1987, at our home.

Throughout this ordeal, I had already passed through much of the grieving process. I was ready for Jim to die, for his suffering to end, and for my life to begin again.

When people ask me how I have maintained my sanity, my reply is always the same: "Faith in God, faith in myself, and a sense of humor!"

As I stated in the introduction, there is no "after AIDS." Once AIDS comes for a visit, it is there to stay. In my own case, I have the memories of Jim's ordeal, as well as my own positive HIV status. When I was tested, I knew in my heart that the results would be positive. After Jim's death, I rested for a brief period of time and then went job hunting in the growing AIDS services industry. I have been doing "AIDS work" ever since—public speaking, counseling and consulting work.

In September of 1988, I was hospitalized with cytomegalovirus (CMV) pneumonia. The fatigue I felt was brutal. Since then, I have been hospitalized three other times for meningitis, severe bronchitis, and intestinal CMV. At the present, I am doing very well, thank God. My saving grace has been my physician,

Larry McDonald, MD, who communicates *with me*, not at me. We make decisions together, as a team would. He listens, and takes a personal interest in my life, my hopes, and my needs.

Many health-care professionals have asked me to tell them some of the things that they can do to help PWAs and their caregivers. I think that the most important things are often overlooked in haste, or for simply the lack of understanding. First and foremost, it is essential that health professionals realize that AIDS is a *chronic illness*. Try to imagine just what these people are experiencing. Whether the person involved is HIV positive, a caregiver, or has full blown AIDS, he is living a life of uncertainty and, often, living for the moment is a necessity. Anyone who is not acquainted with a person living within the realm of HIV infection cannot fully appreciate the incredible problems that these individuals face. Everyday, there may be a new health related, emotional, or financial crisis, and these clients need to be made aware of the full spectrum of possibilities; up front and honestly. Good communication is the key to a successful relationship with the person with AIDS, and his family or significant other. Health professionals, doctors in particular, frequently assume that the general population has a vast education in medicine. Just as AIDS cannot be transmitted by casual contact, neither can education or information. *Talk* to your patients and talk to their families. It can make an enormous difference in the therapeutic relationship. Also, do not assume that the patient is always telling the truth. Jim would tell the doctor that he was feeling fine—no problems—when, actually, he had passed out on the way to the hospital. Take the time to talk to the caregivers, either in person or by telephone, to see if their stories jive with those of the patient.

I became an AIDS expert out of sheer necessity and experience. I read various articles and medical journals to increase my knowledge on the subject. I soon discovered that I knew more than many of the professionals who were working with my husband. Granted, the year was 1986, light years ago in the age of AIDS, but I should not have had to teach myself everything about AIDS. I was dealing with "professionals" and they were getting paid! Again, I must emphasize: *communicate, communicate, communicate.*

Show genuine concern for the family of a person with AIDS; they are going through a tremendous ordeal and are frequently under a great deal of stress. Try to lighten their burden. It is helpful to inform them of little "tricks of the trade" in order to make their life easier. Teach them when it is necessary to wear gloves, how to properly scrub their hands, how to change an Attends, how to make a safe transfer in and out of bed, etc. For example, Jim would be constantly cold right before he became feverish. No matter how many covers I piled on top of him, I could not make him warm. Once a nurse suggested that I place a heating pad near his feet. I tried her little trick and it worked! I never would have thought of that idea on my own.

Encourage caregivers to "take a break" and to do something for *themselves* on a regular basis. Teach the caregivers relaxation techniques, or other stress relievers. Anything to make life a little less hectic will help. Inquire as to if they have enough homecare services, or if they have a family or volunteer support system. Many people do not know that these services exist, and they are so exhausted and stressed out that they do not know where or how to start looking for the necessary assistance. One final thing that one can do to *really* help caregivers is to do little things for them. Don't ask, "What can I do for you?" because there is so much to be done, it may be difficult to come up with one particular chore, or the person may be too embarrassed to ask for help. Instead, say, "Let me go to the store for you, let me do the laundry for you, let me stay with Jim for a few hours while you go out." By taking control, for just a short time, you can allow them to relax a little and to step down from the tightrope; if only for a moment.

A caring touch to a person with AIDS can do more than you know. It tells the person, in a nonverbal way, that you are not afraid of them and that you are genuinely concerned about his or her welfare. The person with AIDS is a human being with human fragilities: he is not a disease. A caring heart is also important. Talk to your patients, find out their feelings. If they become critically ill, what are their wishes? Can you fulfill their needs?

Doctors are trained to save and prolong lives for as long as possible. Quantity of life is important. However, many persons with AIDS are concerned about the *quality* of their lives. For some, it may be enough to sit in bed and gaze out the window at a beautiful day; for others, the idea of being that debilitated is unthinkable. To save and prolong life is a noble cause; however, a person has the right to choose dignity in matters of life and death.

There is still a tremendous amount of ignorance, misconception and misunderstanding about AIDS in the general population, but is also rampant within the medical field, as well. It is very important for people to realize that we are fighting a disease. We are not fighting a person or a lifestyle.

It is also vitally important to realize that AIDS, with the advent of drugs such as azidothymidine (AZT), may be a long-term illness with many ups and downs. It is not unusual for a person to be in the hospital one month, and to be back at work the next month. Life goes on; there are good days and bad days, but people with AIDS are *living* with this disease. People with AIDS should be encouraged to modify behavior, if necessary, to preserve health but, on the other hand, they should try to keep life as normal as possible. Remember, an HIV-positive result or an AIDS diagnosis does not mean that death is coming tomorrow. When a course of proper medical treatment, social and emotional support, diet, personal care, and a positive attitude are followed, life can be meaningful and long-term.

Since Jim's illness, and certainly since his death, my life has changed in ways that I would not even have imagined just a few short years ago; now, it will never be the same. I have a new lifestyle now, a bit different from the last, but for the most part, it is richer and fuller. I know myself better than I ever have before, and I truly like myself. I live my life to the fullest; I have many friends, both old and new, with whom I share good times and sad times. I take each day as it comes and take as much from each day as I possibly can. There are no guarantees in this life, and AIDS will definitely prove it to you.

5 Barry, My Son

Arlene Binkowitz

The Shattering

Deep within the cavernous blackness of the psyche
The shards churn and burn
Illuminating the billions of particles of a tortured being
Piercing, stinging, flailing, choking.
Trying to inhale, but suffocating
From the infinitesimal whirling of the unsettled darkness
That grips the soul.

Deserted of touch, of breath, of smile, of sound,
Denied the love, the promise, the future, the pride.
The intensity of despair can be matched only
With the force and magnitude of immeasurable love
Defined only by another who shares the ultimate shattering
of the human spirit,
The loss of a child, my son, my life.

—Arlene Binkowitz, ©1989

My son, Barry, died on December 18, 1987 at the age of 28.

I finished writing this poem just one year after his death, each word and thought exorcising some of the unbearable pain from my mind and body to the paper on which it was written, each line coveting an insatiable yearning for a son, my only son, whom I will never see again.

Losing a child is undoubtedly the worst tragedy to befall a parent. No one can understand the anguish, the incapacitation, the depression, the ultimate sorrow and sadness engulfing a mother or a father unless they too have lost a child. No one can imagine the abyss of despair the body and mind encounter, nor can you expect anyone else to know. The only solace you seek, your only craving is to hear about your child from those who knew him.

Trying to cope with daily tasks is monumental. Making a cup of coffee or trying to prepare dinner is Herculean. Everyday chores become insurmountable, escape from reality possesses you. I know I speak for anyone who has ever lost a child. The maternal bond of love is so strong and powerful that when you lose a child you have lost a part of your inner self, your soul, your purpose for being.

What I am speaking about is grief. Does it matter that my son died of AIDS? Is society more compassionate to those who have lost a child to an acceptable disease? We lost our son first, that he had AIDS was secondary.

So many parents who have been struck with the devastation of AIDS, and losing a child, have lost not only part of their own lives, but must experience the added stigma of losing a child to a disease that society condemns, a disease that uninformed, ignorant people denounce and force grieving families to hide from and suffer silently.

Perhaps my husband Jerry and I have been more fortunate than many, if such a word exists in our vocabulary today. We have had a wonderful support system of friends and family who have stood by us during Barry's illness and subsequent death, and have given us their hearts and their hands during this shattering year in our lives.

Barry was 28 years old, a second-year resident in psychiatry at St. Vincent's Hospital in New York when he was stricken with this awesome disease. After a grueling four years in Buffalo Medical School, and coming to terms at the same time with his own identity as a gay man, he was thrilled and excited to settle in at Greenwich Village, New York, in a community where he could at last be open and comfortable in his lifestyle, and furthermore be in a hospital where he could fulfill his dreams and ambitions. He embraced his discipline with joy and with triumphant expectations of what his future held for him. In a short time he gained the admiration and respect of his colleagues for his intelligence, his honesty, his astute awareness of human frailties, and his passion for life. He had an innate sensitivity to the human experience and having made well-thought-out decisions and adjustments to his own life, psychiatry was a profession he was well suited for. He loved to tell us stories and anecdotes about his patients, yet with such compassion and understanding of their plight that it was truly amazing to us how he could understand so much about people in so short a time.

During his first year as an intern he was sick several times with a "flu bug" and swollen glands; he had lost weight and was constantly tired. Nonetheless, we attributed these minor illnesses to his first year of residency, which is exhausting and tiring under the best of circumstances, and we did not think much of these episodes except that he was overworked and suffering the stress of all first-year interns.

When he finished his emergency room rotation in May of 1986 he welcomed a vacation to free him from the burdens placed on him during these last months, and he hoped after two weeks he would return to his work with renewed strength and vitality. With two of his friends, he left for Mexico. Less than one week after his departure he called to say he was returning home, too ill to continue his journey. Mother's Day, 1986, he returned home, weak, feverish, and totally debilitated. This was the beginning of our descent into Hell.

Calling on our friends in the medical community we were directed to Dr. Ralph Zalusky, the Chief of Hematology/Oncology at Beth Israel Hospital in New York, whose reputation in the field is unsurpassed. We knew Barry would receive the best treatment available, and subsequently underwent a battery of tests and a biopsy of his lymph glands. Within a week he was diagnosed with Hodgkin's disease, and although in a very advanced stage of the disease, we were bolstered by the fact that Hodgkin's was a curable cancer and he would somehow survive this ordeal. Little did we know then, but were later to learn, was that Barry was HIV-positive, and the combination of Hodgkin's and AIDS would be lethal.

At the outset of his treatment Barry had made a pact with Dr. Zalusky not to tell him if he tested positive to the AIDS virus so that he could cope with the six months of intensive chemotherapy that lay in front of him.

Knowing that Barry was gay, the fear of AIDS was always embedded in our subconscious, but he had always assured us he was careful, and being in the medical and gay community as well, knew more than most about the disease. But there was really not much to know then, except that it was fatal. At that time dealing with the Hodgkin's disease diagnosis was more than enough to bear.

Barry continued to work part-time during his treatment; he was feeling much better, gained back some weight, the fever and chills that he had experienced earlier disappeared and he seemed to be on the road to recovery. His colleagues at St. Vincent's rallied around him and covered for him whenever he was too ill to work, and they gave him tremendous encouragement and support. Throughout his ordeal he maintained a positive, hopeful attitude, refusing to succumb to the despair into which he could easily have fallen, and instead channeled his limited energy into his work.

At the end of the year, just when his chemo treatments were coming to an end, he developed a cough, a cough that eventually led to difficulty in breathing, and he was hospitalized with what was diagnosed as *Pneumocystis carinii* pneumonia (PCP). What was happening to our son was incomprehensible. From having a strong, young, athletic body, he became so weak and fatigued he could hardly stand up. For three weeks he fought the Pneumocystis; we watched a team of physicians streaming in and out of his room, never realizing the seriousness of what was taking place. Barry was well aware that he might be in the realm of AIDS, but he was still hoping this pneumonia was related to the Hodgkin's disease. There was a possibility that after these six long months of intensive chemotherapy he could have developed a pneumonia similar to PCP since his immune system was very much compromised at this point.

Because Barry was a doctor he was accorded the best medical care possible and, with Dr. Zalusky's influence and reputation, everything that could be done for him was. He was also constantly surrounded by friends and family who loved and cared for him, an important factor in his recovery. So many are alone and afraid, ostracized, untouched. Some of the hospital staff would wear gowns and masks just to bring food into the room which left him feeling like a leper. I remember him saying that sometimes one of the nurses would come in and say hello with a smile and hold his hand. That smile didn't take any more effort, but it showed a little caring and compassion. He was a human being, deserving that respect. One cannot get AIDS by touching someone who is ill. I know: I am a mother who has hugged and kissed and cared for her son.

At last he was well enough to go home to recuperate. The day before he was to be discharged from the hospital he noticed a small lesion on his arm, and a biopsy was taken. Nevertheless, we left the hospital feeling joyous; the Hodgkin's was in remission and we would be home for New Year's and would usher in 1987 with our prayers for an end to this nightmare. Little did we know, nothing could be further from the truth.

One week later, just after New Year's, Dr. Zalusky called us all to come into his office. We were so shaken and frightened we could hardly think or move. We clung to each other and held Barry, afraid of what we were about to hear. And then the final blow was delivered. Barry had Kaposi's sarcoma, and this new infection categorized him with full-blown AIDS. Now the true facts were presented to us, and we had to face the realization that Barry might die within the year. But we were still unbelieving. This could not be happening to us, not to our son. We promised Barry we would fight this together, that we would be there for him always, to do for him whatever needed to be done to combat this illness.

I joined a support group of mothers—women whose sons and daughters were diagnosed with AIDS. Most of the mothers had sons who were either gay or had been IV drug users. We shared and bared our pain, our anguish, our fears, yet we gave to each other the support and encouragement we needed to cope, to understand, and to be prepared for the worst. Each of us was in a different stage with our children—some just diagnosed and well, others almost at the end of their lives. We learned about this diabolic illness, the scope of its devastation, the emotional and psychological scars as well as the physical; we witnessed the multitude of opportunistic infections. We shared medical information and drug therapies, and tried to deal with the ignorance and misinformation, with the discrimination and secrecy, with the bureaucratic red tape involved with the myriad of complexities beset by this illness. But most of all we shared our pain, our anger and our frustration, not only for ourselves, but for the children we loved so much and for whom we could do nothing more but hope and pray for time, for a cure, for a new treatment, for tolerance, and at the same time to appreciate the present and to make every moment count.

Barry still worked part-time when he could. He studied and researched and questioned the medical community, became an ardent advocate for self-empowerment. He joined The People with AIDS Coalition, a support group for people with AIDS providing services, information and friendship. Later on, just before he was taken ill in October 1987, he was asked to be the first medical director of the Community Research Initiative, an organization formed within the community to do testing and trials of new AIDS drugs, a place where he would put his efforts and medical training to use while he himself was fighting the battle to survive. He would be in the forefront of new knowledge and one of the first to know about new treatments. It was an exciting new concept and he was prepared to put his abilities to use.

But the Hodgkin's disease returned despite all his efforts to maintain his well-being. He cried like a baby in my arms one day, fearful of the onslaught once again of the chemotherapy. But his doctor assured him that this time the treatment would be less severe—less severe, as we later learned, because his immune system could not tolerate such a battering again. Eventually he would become weaker and weaker, each time a new chemo treatment doing more damage to his already compromised immune system.

Finally, in the Spring of 1987, after another round in the hospital with Hodgkin's, he was forced to take a leave of absence from St. Vincent's, and hoped he would regain his strength without the added stress of working. That summer he swam, he exercised, he ate well and gained weight. He was with his friends and family as much as possible. He looked wonderful, and we thought, "maybe he will be the one to beat this disease, and maybe some new treatment will be found soon, and he will make it." I know that every mother who is caring for a child with AIDS is thinking these same thoughts. After peaking to an incredible high, feeling better than ever, his body gave out once again, and he was hospitalized with the return of the Hodgkin's disease and another dose of chemotherapy.

During his next to the last stay in the hospital, several weeks before he died, I stayed overnight with him in his room. We spoke of many things that night—of life, of death, of his memorial. Barry felt he had lived life to the fullest in his 28 years, and that despite his illness this last year was the best he ever had. He learned the true value of his friendships—friendships of unconditional love and support. He understood the importance and meaning of life—a life he led, rich and replete, fuller than most people would have if they lived to be many more years than he. The only discomfort he felt was the pain of those who loved him—those who would miss him so when he was gone. He believed he was here on a mission, he said, and soon he would be embarking on a new adventure. "How can you say that," I asked him, "when your whole future and medical career are ahead of you. There is so much you haven't done, so much you haven't seen." He replied by saying that he did everything he wanted to do, and the only thing left to do would be more of the same.

With these thoughts in mind, I found the following words he had written within the last few months before his death: "I am filled and absolutely fulfilled on all levels as a human being, and am eternally thankful for this life."

In December 1987, Barry went into the hospital for the last time.

How do you prepare for the death of your 28-year-old son whose whole promising future lies ahead of him? How can you believe living in the 1980s there is an incurable disease with no drugs or treatment available to make him well, that no effort has been made in seven years to stem its escalation or find a cure. When do you think you will wake up and find this is not really happening?

Many parents are ashamed and humiliated at the stigma attached to this illness. Fathers, especially, have turned away from their children. So many have died without their parents near, without their love, their support, their acceptance. I have been fortunate that my husband has always been supportive, loving and caring. His primary concern was Barry's health, and he was there whenever he needed him.

The pride we have felt for our son, his accomplishments, his dignity, his compassion, his honesty, his love, his humor, his philosophy of life—those are the attributes that characterized him as a human being. Our love and support for him never diminished because he was gay. The most important thing to him was knowing that we still loved and accepted him, and we did. He didn't choose to be gay. He was.

I read somewhere that in a field of common poppies a wildflower grows, beautiful and distinct among the ordinary, but nonetheless beautiful. My son was one of those special flowers. Time and again since his death we have been told by his friends and colleagues about the inspiration and spirit he instilled in them with his determination and courage. He seemed to possess an inner strength and serenity uncommon in a person so young. He touched the lives of everyone he met.

One friend wrote to us after he learned of Barry's death, terribly distressed that he was away when Barry died. It was only after repeated phone calls to his apartment without an answer that he knew something was ominously wrong. In a letter to us he wrote:

> Don't let anyone take your grief away from you. It is yours, and even for each of you it is different. Live with it and live through it in your own way. But also keep in touch with Barry, not only as the son you desperately long for, but also as the son who will always live within you, closer to you than any longing or words or thoughts or tears. Don't separate him from you by only longing for him. Keep him even closer to you, within you, because experiencing his love for you, more than anything else, can help you. Keep open to his love and his light. I cannot remember ever having met anyone who loved his parents more than Barry.

Instances like these with so many of his friends and colleagues have kept his spirit alive in our hearts and have brought comfort to us in this time of utter despair and frustration.

Our family has never followed religion in any ritualistic sense. We join the Jewish people in prayer during the high holy days and have always taken part as a family in celebrating all the important and festive holidays. Barry was always a part of these festivities and he looked forward to being with the family on these special occasions. He went to Israel for a college semester and spent six months at Tel Aviv University. Meeting our Israeli family for the first time, he became one of them, learning the language, exploring the country, being part of the tradition and heritage he was brought up with. He loved the country so much that he chose to do a rotation there during medical school. Our Israeli family treated him as if he were their own son. Twenty-eight trees have been planted in the hills of Jerusalem to commemorate his death, to remember him, and to enrich the beauty of the land.

Barry's acceptance of God was written in some random notes I found after he had died. It seems that at this point in his illness he was reaching for a spiritual meaning to life, and was trying to comprehend death and its consequences. In his journal, he wrote:

> The first premise is to accept the idea that we are all-loving and that love is the energy of life-force.
> The second premise is the acknowledgement that in each of us is God. And we can each define that uniquely. For me then, God is all knowing and all-loving. And therefore, if God lies within each of us, then each of us has within all-knowledge and all loving. Then, each of us has within all knowledge and pure love, so that everything we need to know is within ourselves. And so then, if all the answers lie within we must find the paths to our inner selves, our higher selves.
> Now, let us assume that each of us, as human beings, has the ability to reach our higher selves, the God within us. It is then that we are in touch with the higher human consciousness, with the reservoir of all that is known, has been known and will be known, and the pure radiant energy of love.

Barry would have made a wonderful doctor with his natural sensitivity, with his ability to understand human suffering from his own experience with Hodgkin's disease, with his compassion and love, with his zest for life. As parents we have lost his future and all it represents, the pride, the promise, the fulfillment of our years, the perpetuation of our own lives. An obituary written by one of our friends stated: "Society's loss of a uniquely gifted physician at the threshold is profound."

Just before Barry entered the hospital in December 1987, he had experienced severe pain in the area of his kidneys, but he hoped that this was just another infection that could be treated with antibiotics. Once in the hospital, tests were ordered and various medications were given to him to reduce his pain and the swelling of his now bloated body. Everything proved negative. Once more the Hodgkin's disease reared its ugly head, and yet another different chemotherapy was tried. Barry knew that no one could tolerate the amount of chemotherapy his body had already ingested all these months and still survive. But his incorruptible faith in Dr. Zalusky always sustained him and gave him hope. This time the doctor was attending a conference out of town for several days and could not be with Barry at this grave time. His rapport with the other doctors, although friendly and considerate, was not the same as with Dr. Z. He patiently awaited his return to see what ideas he had up his sleeve.

Barry and Dr. Zalusky had a very special relationship, one of mutual sharing, confidence and trust, one not only of patient and doctor, but of partners and colleagues. He admired Barry's insight and perception, his optimism, the mental and physical challenge under which he accepted this illness. Barry, in turn, totally trusted the doctor's judgment, his astuteness, his resourcefulness, his knowledge, and his ability in treating him. Together, they carefully discussed his treatment, its effects and its progression before formulating the best route to take. Whatever they decided was done as a team, each giving to the other the resolve and truth to face reality, neither ever losing hope, but always aware of the strong possibility of death.

When the doctor returned from his trip he called us immediately, and very protectively and compassionately told us that this time Barry would not be leaving the hospital, and that we must make every effort to make his last days comfortable, hopeful and free of pain.

I listened in complete disbelief, my mind not hearing the words of finality, that death was so near. The world floated by, the breath of my body collapsing within me. I tried to concentrate on the immediate. Still in my office, I had to make arrangements to leave, not knowing when I would return. Jerry and I would remain with Barry in the hospital until the end.

I remember functioning in a haze, not really comprehending anything I was saying or doing. One of my friends at the office accompanied me to the hospital. I was too panicked to be on my own.

We never expected this trip to the hospital to be one of such sudden gravity. Although Barry had grown weaker in the last two months with several hospital stays, he was always in good spirits, overcoming obstacles, pushing himself to the limits of his existence. But though we knew he might be facing death, it is really not a tangible idea; you can never believe your child is going to die. It is an impossible thought; you can talk about it, think about it, anticipate it, but not really expect it is ever going to happen.

Dr. Zalusky was waiting for us in the hospital lounge. Facing the truth was still unimaginable, but coming from the person in whose hands our son's life rested, and whose unerring judgment we trusted more than anyone else's, the words finally brought us back to earth. The Hodgkin's disease was in his liver. It was only a matter of time now. No heroics would be performed, no unnecessary pain suffered, everything would be done for him that was humanly possible to make him comfortable.

Dazed and incredulous, we somehow managed to ask the doctor if he would give the eulogy at Barry's funeral. Without hesitation he agreed and said it would be his honor to do so. Giving a eulogy for a patient is almost unheard of in the medical community, but their relationship was a special one, and speaking for Barry was almost as if he were speaking for his own son.

During the next two weeks in the hospital, we rallied the support of all Barry's friends, colleagues and our family and friends. We actually took over the lounge on the hospital floor where Barry's room was, even giving out the public phone number there to anyone who needed to reach us so that we would not disturb Barry in his room with phone calls.

All day and every day for more than ten days the waiting room took on not a somber atmosphere, but rather one of togetherness, support and confidence. Friends and family came from California, Philadelphia, Chicago, Florida, Provincetown, every one of them taking a turn to see him. Some sat for hours for a glimpse or a word with him, or just a smile. There was a steady stream of visitors from early in the morning until late at night. Sometimes there were 30 or more people in the lounge at one time just waiting to see him, buoying our spirits as well as Barry's. It was truly an outpouring of enormous dedication and love from everyone who knew him.

And then the last day. He was still hopeful and waiting to go home. That morning he told my husband he felt he needed some exercise. Being bedridden for so many days he felt the need to stretch his legs. My husband helped him move his legs up and down to provide better circulation and to make him more comfortable. That afternoon he took his last breath, quietly and peacefully with my husband and me at his side.

On a rainy, cold day in December 1987, four hundred people gathered to pay tribute to my son at his funeral.

In the Jewish religion, there is a period of *shiva* after the funeral which lasts for several days. Visitors and friends come to pay their condolences, to help ease the sorrow. Our home was filled with people day and night trying to help us get through the worst time in our lives.

Our friends have been a truly significant force in our survival, enduring friendships that have proven to us again the meaning of unconditional love. In time of crisis, they have given of their time unselfishly, attended to our needs, listed to our sorrow, and have been there for us whenever we needed them. Each in his or her own way has provided us with a means of being in the present. And each has continued to express his or her concern. Yes, we have been most fortunate.

I returned to my job as soon as I could after Barry died. Keeping busy is one's salvation. Tears can continually flow, their supply inexhaustible. Reminiscences, covering every facet of his being, pop in and out of my consciousness; leaving me in constant torment. Working helps to alleviate some of the incessant, gnawing pain. My co-workers are people I've worked with for more than 25 years in a job that has been a second family to me. Everyone has given me the space and time to breathe and allowed me the freedom to grieve at my own pace without pressure and imposition. I have been more than grateful for all their support, kindness and compassion in the wake of this awesome tragedy.

My mother, on the other hand, could not cope with the loss of her grandson. It was too much for her to bear. Her heart was broken, her life no longer had any meaning. She had been with us from dawn to midnight every day during the long vigil in the hospital. When Barry died I believe her life actually ended, maybe not physically, but within her soul. Wendy, my daughter, and Barry were her precious jewels, her reason for living. She adored them, as they did her.

After Barry died I could not grieve with her because my own pain was too severe. Yet I knew how desperately lost she was facing this sorrow. The pain of carrying her grief along with mine was unrelenting, and so I ignored hers and tried to show her how well I was coping. But deep within that "cavernous psyche" I wished that she would not suffer so. It was more pain than she had to endure her entire life.

Only three months after Barry's death she developed a brain tumor which caused her to hemorrhage and go into a coma, a coma from which she never recovered. And so another vigil began, ironically in the same hospital where Barry had been. Each day we opened the same doors, walked along the same corridors, saw some of the same nurses. At the end, with my daughter at her side, singing to her, telling her it was all right to let go and be with Barry, she quietly and peacefully left this world in the hopes perhaps of joining her grandson in a new life.

There I was again, faced with yet another death. My mother, 76 years old, my son, 28. I could not mourn my mother that first year. My sensibilities were at the depths of such despair already there was no room for more grief. It is only now, one year later, that I try to look back and remember her. Yet, it is still difficult to realize the full extent of her death, or feel the real pain. After all, one does not expect your child to die before your mother. It is not in the natural order of life. I still cannot believe she is really gone. How can I? When I still cannot believe my son is dead, and that I will never see either of them again.

In the aftermath of these tragedies, my husband and I have tried to survive by keeping Barry's memory alive, by feeling his presence always around us. We even sought out a psychic hoping to hear a message "from the other side"—to be in touch with his spirit and light. The desperate need to believe in an afterlife consumes you for a time. It gives you something to cling to, as if you could still be with him for a while longer.

In reality, we have tried to rebuild our lives out of the chaos and to create new meaning for ourselves. As never before, we are learning the lessons of both my son and my mother to value every precious moment of life, to enjoy the present—for tomorrow is the unexpected, the unknown.

Bereavement counseling is by far the most important step in taking control of your life after a death, especially of a child. Coping with the stigma of AIDS complicates ordinary counseling one might seek. It is an additional issue to be addressed, and finding the right person or group to help you is a must for your mental health.

I was referred by a friend to a bereavement counselor, Rosemarie Ampela, whom I began to see soon after my mother died. Within weeks my husband too started therapy sessions with her. Mere words cannot express our gratitude to her. Without her help this year we may never have been able to withstand the power of our grief. She has taken us from the darkness into the light, and has guided us to the good and positive things still in our lives.

It is amazing how insightful she has been in learning about Barry from us. Often she will tell us how Barry might have reacted in a situation and why he accepted life's challenges with such courage. It is almost as if she herself knew him, and has showed us a part of him that we never fully recognized as an adult. But most importantly, she has impressed on us how much Barry loved us, and how much our love meant to him.

During his last days in the hospital I promised Barry we would have a memorial for him. He wanted to have a celebration of his life, a place where his friends and family would gather to speak about him and have a good time. He visualized the day with a grin on his face, and a light in his eyes.

In June 1988, six months after his death, we did have a celebration for him. St. Vincent's Hospital extended their hospitality to us, and with the talents of their extraordinary staff, they provided us with a place for Barry's Celebration of Life. In a room filled with flowers, balloons, beautiful decorations, and a delectable buffet, 150 people gathered to honor him and celebrate with us. What a momentous day that was. I think it was truly what Barry had envisioned. This day, our hearts were filled with pride and joy instead of sadness and pain.

The staff, the doctors at St. Vincent's, his friends and our family came to be a part of that day. They spoke about him, laughed about him, honored him. My daughter sang a beautiful song for which she had composed the lyrics and melody. Unknown to us, while Barry was in the hospital she sang the uncompleted version to him and promised him it would be finished by the time of his memorial. In a hushed room everyone listened, cried and applauded. She was the highlight of the afternoon. It was a day we will always remember, and I believe everyone who was there with us will remember as well.

My husband and I planned to dedicate a room in St. Vincent's in Barry's name, and on that day the honor was bestowed on him. A plaque was placed outside the Rounds Room in the Psychiatric Ward, the room where he would begin his work each day, where the doctors meet each morning before they see their patients. It was a special place for him, and it is now a special place for us, and the staff of St. Vincent's.

Along with our own personal response to Barry's death, we have helped to raise money for AIDS organizations of which Barry had been a part, The People with AIDS Coalition and the Community Research Initiative (CRI) in New York. The Clinical Trials Floor at the CRI was dedicated in his name and a plaque hangs on the wall with his picture. Panels have been made for him at the NAMES Project by his friends, and we too have volunteered our time both in New York and Washington.

Writing has become a form of therapy for me. I started a journal after Barry died and have continued with it to now. Though I have a formidable support system and an exceptional husband always at my side, I cannot escape the loneliness and desolation within my soul. In a crowded room of people, I am very much alone with that pain. Writing has been a cathartic for some of that pain, and since Barry's death I have written some poetry, and a story about my mother which has been published in *Bereavement Magazine*, a marvelous journal of hope and healing. I have spoken at the dedications to Barry, and just recently addressed the New York Board of Rabbis about our personal experience, to awaken the consciousness of the Jewish community to the ravages of this illness. And now I have been privileged to write this chapter, to continue to reach out to others and to rekindle the flame of Barry's memory.

Barry, too, reached out to the AIDS community while he was alive. Many of his wishes have been achieved. When the first discussions of "underground" drugs were brought to the AIDS community, Barry was among the first, questioning, investigating, learning as much as he could about the effects of new drugs and treatments. He was one of the principal recipients of a food substance of egg lipids, or AL721, which he advocated using. He strongly recommended the use of aerosol pentamidine, a very promising preventative for PCP which was being used by only a few doctors knowledgeable enough to understand its performance and effects on people with AIDS. One of these physicians, Dr. Joseph Sonnabend, a tireless, dedicated physician, was working with AIDS patients at the very beginning of the outbreak and saw the drug's potential in its early development. Even Barry's own private physicians were not sanctioning its use, but Barry believed that one day it would prove advantageous in preventing the onset of PCP. The Food and Drug Administration (FDA) has since approved its use as a new AIDS treatment.

Proper nutrition, vitamins and exercise were part of the daily regimen in maintaining his health. Yoga, creative visualization and meditation were also part of the program he practiced in nursing his body. Keeping a positive, hopeful frame of mind throughout surely prolonged his life, if only for a short time. He was determined to nurture his body with whatever means he could as long as they were safe and compatible with his own medications; he did everything he could to sustain his life.

When he was well enough during the year, he visited his cousin, Rita, a poet and writer, who lives in Provincetown. The tranquility of the small town off-season, the smell of the sea air, the total caring environment she provided him, enabled him to see life clearly and in harmony with his own existence. He joined in bringing the AIDS community there the knowledge of his own experiences, sources of new drugs and treatment, and the great importance of self-empowerment in fighting this battle.

Last year when we visited my cousin during the summer, people from the town came to meet us as Barry's parents, to let us know how significant his contribution was, and still is, to the people with AIDS in Provincetown and how his legacy and essence live on.

As a result of his persistence, and her commitment and promise to him, my cousin founded Provincetown Positive/PWA Coalition which in large measure was due to Barry's foresight. She has brought a world of information to the community, and with the help and support of her many devoted friends who knew and loved Barry as well, has established one of the most aggressive, accomplished and active coalitions in the country.

With the wonderful support of our friends and family during this shattering year, with Barry's friends as well, who are very much a part of our life, with my daughter who has helped us to see Barry's inner light and spirituality, and with the guidance of an extraordinary therapist throughout this year, we have been able to cope with our devastating loss. There is not a moment in the day that we do not think of him, what he was, what he could have been. There will always be a void in our lives without him.

Words in his own journal underscore his realization of the magnitude of this illness. He wrote: "We must understand that we all have AIDS, every man, woman and child; that we all have AIDS in our consciousness, and that we must work together as a human community against this disease."

There is the promise of hope on the horizon. As my son did, we must live with that hope and pass it on to those people living with AIDS, with the respect and dignity they are entitled to as human beings.

Reflecting on Barry's life, we know that his message to others would be—never to give up hope, treasure every moment of your life, and give love unconditionally. If we can reach into the consciousness of other parents and people to love and accept their children and their fellow human beings unconditionally, to reach into every community to strengthen the bonds of family no matter what the circumstances, to become aware of the dimensions of this illness, which is infiltrating every race, religion, occupation and profession, every economic strata, and to overcome fear, intolerance and discrimination, then perhaps our son, and all those who have died, will not have died in vain.

6 Children and AIDS

Mary Tasker, MSW

Rachel weeping for her children, and would not be comforted because they are not.

—Jeremiah 31:15

Introduction

It was early September 1987. Lucia was on time, as usual, for her clinic appointment. She was accompanied by her aunt, Maria. This was not unusual. Maria had come with the child on previous dates when her sister, Carmen, Lucia's mother, was not feeling well. Lucia looked as radiant as ever. She was a physically beautiful child. Her lustrous hair was brushed to a radiant, dark chestnut sheen. Perhaps she was a little quieter than usual; it was difficult to say. Perhaps we had not expected her to come. It had been just two weeks since her mother died of AIDS. But then she had also kept her clinic appointment 12 days after her baby brother, Carlos, had died of AIDS. That had been only four months ago. Two years before, her father, Roberto, had died of AIDS.

Of the 2,258 children diagnosed with AIDS in the United States as of April 30, 1990, approximately 80 percent have a parent with, or at risk for, HIV infection.[1] Clearly then, to speak of the child with AIDS is almost, by definition, to speak of the family with AIDS. The issues are inseparable.

At the present time pediatric AIDS is over-represented in the minority communities. Black children constitute 15 percent of the nation's children, but 53 percent of all childhood AIDS cases. Hispanic children, who represent 10 percent of the population of U.S. children, account for 22 percent of all childhood AIDS cases.[1] This chapter therefore focuses on the issues confronting the families of children with AIDS as represented by two minority families: Carmen's, of Puerto Rican origin, and a Black family headed by Doris.

Case Histories of Two Families: Doris and Carmen

Doris' Family

Doris is the legal guardian and maternal grandmother of six-year old Tenisha and three-year-old Shantell, who are sisters. The two girls have lived with Doris for almost three years, since Shantell's birth. Their mother, Evelyn, Doris' second-youngest daughter, had fled the hospital soon after giving birth to Shantell, leaving the child behind. Evelyn was an active IV drug user at the height of her disease (drug addiction). She called Doris from a pay phone and begged her to keep Tenisha and Shantell until "I can get this monkey off my back."

Shortly after Evelyn had called Doris from a pay phone, Doris was called by the hospital where Shantell had been born and asked to come and meet with the doctors who were concerned about Shantell's health. They told her that Evelyn had consented to have some tests performed on Shantell before she left the hospital. It appeared that the baby was very underdeveloped and had some kind of lung infection.

Doris recalled that after she recovered from the shock that hit her when she first heard the word AIDS connected to Shantell, her next reaction was disbelief to the point of incredulity. Doris was under the impression that it was "only gay men who got AIDS, and also those drug people who use needles." Certainly Shantell did not fit into either of these categories.

Then the doctor told her that the babies of people who had used drugs also got the AIDS virus. As Doris was about to protest that her daughter, Evelyn, had "never messed around with needles," another blinding flash hit Doris: the difficult time she had experienced with Evelyn through her adolescence; her daughter's truancy from school; the drastic and sudden mood swings she had endured; the many times money had seemed to disappear from the household. Doris turned to look over her shoulder at Evelyn, who had reluctantly accompanied her and knew then what she had denied all those years: her daughter was a drug addict.

Carmen's Family

Though many families first learn of the AIDS diagnosis through the identification of an infected child, Carmen had a somewhat different experience. Carmen had been separated from her husband for two years when he became terminally ill. She says she took him back into her home because he was dying and "someone had to take care of him, after all, he is the father of my children." Carmen did not know why her husband was dying, though she suspected it had something to do with his drug use over many years. It was only after his death that she heard whispers in the community that he had died of AIDS. At first, Carmen was inclined to ignore the rumors; but the more she looked at her younger child, Carlos, who was so small and frail for his age, who had been sick so often, the more afraid she grew.

Finally, she took the children to a nearby hospital where she had heard there was a doctor who worked with children with AIDS. Carmen told herself she was really taking them to clear up her own mind and to prove to the gossiping neighbors what fools they were. After all, Carlos had never actually had to stay in the hospital, and Lucia—well, it was crazy to even think about Lucia being sick. She was the most beautiful child in the family and had just finished first grade.

Carmen walked home from the hospital after hearing that both of her children were infected with the AIDS virus. She needed to clear her mind and regain control. As she watched her two children holding hands on the way home, she noted the features they had inherited from her. Carlos was very small with the biggest brown eyes you had ever seen; Lucia had the same beautiful, thick hair that Carmen had been so vain about in herself as an adolescent.

As they turned the corner to their street, Carmen could see up ahead the entrance to the local funeral parlor. As she thought of this other terrible legacy her children had "inherited" from her—AIDS—she wondered how long it would be before she might have to enter those doors. Carmen felt an incredible wave of nausea sweep over her: of anger toward her husband, but, even more, of hatred toward herself. She said to herself, "I knew he was a bad man; I knew he was doing those drugs. I knew I had no right to call myself a good mother for having babies with that man. It's my fault, it's my fault my children got the AIDS. If my babies die, it will be all my fault."

The guilt feelings experienced by Carmen as she saw herself as the cause of her children's imminent deaths were also experienced in another way by Doris. Doris felt guilt over raising a child who had become a drug addict, who, in turn, had given birth to a child who now had AIDS. Later in the course of Shantell's illness, she said, the nurses "were talking to me about how all the mothers feel so guilty having given AIDS to their kids. How do they think I feel? I'm the one that's responsible for two generations having AIDS."

The Diagnosis is Revealed

The day a child is diagnosed as being HIV/AIDS infected is one that is indelibly etched in the mind of the child's parent (guardian, caregiver). Parents recall the time they first heard "that word" being stated in connection with their child as the day their world stood still.

Doris: "When that doctor told me Shantell was sick because she had the AIDS virus, it was like a thunderbolt struck through me and turned me to stone. I was deaf, dumb, and blind all at the same time."

Carmen: "All of a sudden it came to me that she was telling *me* that my baby had the AIDS virus. After she said that word, I believe I couldn't hear another thing she was saying, though I'm sure she was still talking because her mouth was still moving."

The shock and horror experienced by parents at this time appears to cause an invisible wall to arise and surround the family, a wall that protects as it shuts out the terrifying new knowledge. This "wall" experience seems to provide a buffer against the immediate impact of hearing the diagnosis for the first time.

For a family to discover through the diagnosis of a child that HIV/AIDS endangers the welfare of the whole family, is not an unusual experience. The symptoms of pediatric HIV infection often manifest themselves much earlier in a child, whose immune system is not yet fully matured.[2]

Guilt and Stigma: To Tell or Not to Tell

An air of secrecy is often the cloak that accompanies a diagnosis of AIDS, for a child as well as an adult. To reveal that a child has AIDS is to automatically raise the question of how the child became infected and, inevitably, to bring to light the "behaviors" that led to infection by the virus. Gay men already had much sad experience with stigma before AIDS. Minorities felt stigma attached to them due to language or pigmentation. AIDS added to that burden. The term "coming out of the closet" was coined by gays prior to the advent of AIDS. The issue of telling or not telling, secrecy or openness, lying or truthfulness, is an inner struggle common to all PWAs. For most parents of children with AIDS, the issue usually becomes not only one of *if* to tell, but eventually who, when, how, and how much to tell.

For two years Doris would decide to keep Shantell's diagnosis to herself, thus, she felt, avoiding any possibility of the secret becoming known either within or outside of the family. Doris would say that she felt the most concerned because of Tenisha, Shantell's sister. Tenisha did not carry the virus and would therefore be able to enjoy a normal life, going to school and having friends. If the diagnosis became known, Tenisha might be subject to the rejection and isolation often inflicted, not only on PWAs, but also on anyone closely associated with them. Thus the secrecy issue, while protecting Tenisha from the harmful effects of stigma, also meant that Doris would have to suffer the burden alone and unsupported.

In Carmen's case her initial reluctance to reveal the secret to anyone else was connected not only to her fear of stigma for her children and herself, but also because she did not want to reveal to the world that she had been married to a drug addict. She particularly felt the need to conceal this fact from her father, who, she stated, had warned her many times not to marry Roberto because he was "no good." Carmen confided to her social worker, "How do you think my father will react to me when he finds out he was right? How do you think I feel? Maybe this is the punishment I get for disobeying my father's advice." The feeling of being punished for wrongdoing has been described by many professionals working with families.[3]

Telling Children Their Diagnosis

With regard to the questions of telling, children are often completely left out of this debate. Professionals working with families of children with AIDS are themselves very divided on this issue. While the literature on chronic illness in children abounds with advocates who believe that children should know their diagnosis, the debate still rages in pediatric AIDS whether the word AIDS should ever be mentioned to a child, given the strength and power of the stigma attached to that word. While these positions have merit, they entirely overlook the fact that a child may come to know his diagnosis regardless of whether the child is told or not.

Of our two families, Carmen was the first to decide to talk openly about the diagnosis of AIDS, not only to family and outsiders, but also to her daughter Lucia. Carmen's way of telling Lucia this important information was consistent with the ways she always imparted critical knowledge to her daughter. She would think about the issue for a long period of time, mull it over with her most trusted sister Maria, then eventually call Lucia to her side in a quiet moment and present the facts to her. As always, with matters of such importance, Lucia was instructed that these were private family matters, not to be discussed with anyone unless her mother gave approval. So accustomed was Lucia to this mode of operating, that even after coming to clinic for over one year and meeting with her social worker for play therapy sessions, she never acknowledged that she had been told her diagnosis until she was instructed by her mother that she could do so.

While Doris eventually came to share the diagnosis with some members of her family, she was adamant that Shantell and Tenisha should never hear the word AIDS. While Shantell was very young, Tenisha was already in school and had a lively imagination and an inquiring spirit. Tenisha was used to having her questions answered, but it often seemed to her that there were too many questions unanswered. Why was Shantell sick all the time? Why did she have to stay in the hospital so long? Why didn't Mommy live with them or at least visit more often? Why was Grandma Doris angry with Mommy when she did come to visit? Why did Mommy act like she was drunk sometimes? In fact, Doris was not able to talk to Tenisha about the AIDS diagnosis until over a year *after* Shantell had died. Through the therapeutic benefits she derived from a post-bereavement counseling group, Doris was eventually able to talk to Tenisha, not only about the cause of her sister's death, but also about Mommy's drug problem, which Doris was now able to recognize as an illness and not a moral failing on either Evelyn's or her own part.

Therapeutic Work with Children with AIDS

My own professional bias is that children should know the name of their diagnosis at the earliest date; nevertheless, much therapeutic work can be done with children regardless of whether they know their diagnosis or not.

Children of all ages respond to picture and story books, especially when seated close to a parent or another adult they trust and care for. In the waiting room of a busy clinic, as children arrive for their monthly infusions of IV gamma globulin, the tedious and inevitable waiting can be eased if children are read to. In my own work with children in this setting, I would greet the children as they arrived, and they would become familiar with the routine of choosing one of the special books I would present to them. Among the ten or so books always offered, two books were selected far more frequently than all the others. One was a book about visiting a doctor or clinic; the other dealt with a child's fear of nightmares and monsters.

The "doctor" book, as it came to be called, dealt with the very concrete issues that the children would be faced with in the course of the clinic visit. It pictured children in clinic waiting rooms along with the various instruments used by the nurses and doctors, the routine of the clinic visit, and, eventually, the child going home with the parent. Children of all ages responded to the book. The youngest children who were in early verbal stages of naming objects in their world would demonstrate the use of any object they could not name. This was facilitated by also presenting, for their play, a toy doctor kit. Thus, in play, children acted out the very real experiences they would encounter.

The monster book was another favorite. During the course of the two years I worked at this hospital, I photocopied dozens of copies of this book for parents to take home to read to their children. Once again the book appealed to a wide age group. What child could not relate to a little boy's fear of monsters and, in this story, his ability to eventually conquer that fear? Children most probably related to the fear on both a concrete level (fear of the needle), and a more abstract level (fear of death).

Therapeutic Work During Hospitalization

Shantell was an inpatient for many months and, like so many of the children, became so familiar with the routine of the medical setting that any deviation in, for example, a routine physical examination was met with either cries of protest or howls of derision that it was "being done wrong." During the later months of her hospital stay, Shantell suffered from unrelenting abdominal pain that eventually caused her to lose all interest in play. In an effort to lessen the monotony of her hospital room, play sessions were established for Shantell twice a week. Though she was never able to play for very long, Shantell alternated her play between two arenas. One was the play kitchen. On less painful days Shantell happily cooked pancakes for me ("Gwamma do this for my bweakfast"), a reflection of her memory and longing for home.

The other arena was the "hospital," equipped with a toy medical kit, dolls, bottles, blankets and crib. On days when her pain and discomfort overcame the effects of her medication, the baby doll was given a thorough physical examination by "Dr. Shantell," always concluding with the supreme moment when the shot in the arm was given. On days when Shantell needed to be more in touch with her feelings about the medical regimen, the needle part of the routine would be performed on me. I "learned" my role from Shantell, asking her, "How will it feel?" Depending on her mood, Shantell would tell me it would hurt a lot or it would not. Thus, under her direction I would act out the appropriate response. Sometimes I would yell and curse and act out, to which Shantell would respond with great glee. If I was so "directed," I would exhibit fear and cry very sadly, and would, in turn, be comforted by Shantell. She was directing and setting the stage in order to re-experience her fears and other feelings, thus learning to cope with them in an environment over which she felt more control.

When Parent and Child are Hospitalized at the Same Time

We are most keenly aware that pediatric AIDS is AIDS in the family when a parent and child are hospitalized over the same time period. This is not an unusual occurrence in the lives of these families. During one of Carlos's infrequent hospitalizations, his mother, a daily visitor to the child, became seriously ill and also required admitting to a nearby hospital.

This situation gives rise to many complications for the families, both practical and emotional. If there are siblings in the family, who will care for them? If, as in Carmen's family, another member has the virus and becomes ill, who will care for that person or escort them to regular clinic appointments? What about the psychological implications for parent and child concerning separation and isolation? Carlos barely tolerated the separation from Carmen when she had to return home to care for Lucia: her total absence would deepen Carlos's terrible anguish. These situations become doubly complicated if the secret of the diagnosis is still being kept within the family circle. Fortunately, in the case of Carmen's family, the diagnosis had been shared with family members. Thus, Carmen could turn to her family for assistance, consistent with the cultural norms of families of Puerto Rican origin.[4] Creative ways to help lessen the emotional pain of the separation could include the use of taped messages between parent and child. One parent made a tape for her child that included familiar songs and stories. Another parent, who had advance warning of her own hospitalization, brought a Polaroid camera to her child's hospital room and asked the staff to take pictures of her with her child in her arms. She then distributed several of these photographs to the child's primary nurse and social worker, requesting they show the photograph to the child during each professional encounter. They came to think of this photograph as their "passport" to the child, authorizing them to represent the mother during the hospitalization.

When a Parent's Death Precedes a Child's

Since Elizabeth Kubler-Ross's *On Death and Dying* was first published, the literature on working with the terminally ill adult and child has grown tremendously. However, the unique aspect of pediatric AIDS, which is to say AIDS in the family, calls for a new literature which has not yet been written. Like all sound theory, the literature should come first from experience and the reflection on that experience. One could wish that we would never gain sufficient experience from which to cull a theory and hence a literature. Yet AIDS among children one to four years of age is now the ninth leading cause of death and, if current trends continue, could rise to become one of the five leading causes of death within the next three or four years.[1] While awaiting that literature, professionals who are working with families with AIDS at the present time therefore have an obligation to share their experiences, knowledge and skills immediately and frequently.

I have observed that a parent who is dying is reluctant to deal with his own feelings about impending death until the work of making arrangements for the care of surviving children has first been resolved. Parental concern for the care and well-being of a child after their own death is often expressed more directly to professionals than any other single issue. My own experience is that parents have responded well to the introduction of the topic by trusted professionals, when they have been unable to broach it themselves.

Carmen had postponed this topic prior to her youngest child's death, but as she herself become more feeble, she became more keenly aware of her need to provide for continuity in Lucia's life. Carmen feared that her death might be followed by a battle for custody over Lucia between her own family and that of her ex- and now deceased husband. Several months prior to her death, Carmen was encouraged to discuss the issue with her mother, her sister Maria, and her social worker. Maria and Carmen formulated a plan whereby the two sisters became joint legal guardians of the child immediately. Additionally, a will was drawn up which stated Carmen's desire that, on her death, Maria should become sole legal guardian of Lucia. Once this was accomplished, Carmen began to occasionally join a support group to talk about her own fears of her approaching death.

When a Child's Death Precedes a Parent's

Throughout Shantell's final hospitalization, indeed, throughout her short life, Doris had been her legal guardian and sole caretaker. Shantell's mother, Evelyn, visited the child episodically and usually on the urging of Doris. As the child began to fail, Evelyn visited the hospital more frequently but stayed in her daughter's room for shorter periods of time each visit. Often she visited the hospital and never entered the child's room at all. At these times she would spend increasing amounts of time talking with other parents of children with AIDS, "helping to comfort them," she explained to those who chose to challenge her behavior. The professional staff could never adequately reach Evelyn's ambivalence and sense of powerlessness and guilt. Evelyn, always an active drug user, coped with her feelings by increasing her drug-using activities and eventually coming to the hospital high. Doris, angry and ashamed of her daughter, would then throw Evelyn out of Shantell's room, and thus Evelyn accomplished what she desperately sought, a legitimate "reason" not to visit the child.

Doris turned more actively to her spiritual and religious roots in order to cope with Shantell's impending death. Doris spent many hours reading her Bible, sometimes sharing passages she felt spoke to her pain and ease it. Other times she would sit quietly introspective, yet seemed to enjoy regular contact with those professionals she had grown to trust, especially if they were able to understand that sometimes their mere physical presence or companionship was sufficient.

Many times I would save my visits to Shantell's room until the end of the regular work day. I would go and sit with Doris as the child slept in her arms. The silence of those times, though sometimes fraught with a heavy sorrow, brought comfort to us both where words could not. Doris taught me to be at peace with that, for which I will always be in her debt.

We began our story, and thus this chapter's journey, with Lucia's clinic visit shortly after her mother's death, and so we conclude with that same clinic visit. Responding to what I perceived to be Lucia's desire to achieve continuity through the familiar routine, I presented the choice of books to her and she made several selections. Conspicuously absent from her initial selection, was the book dealing with the death of a relative. I read to Lucia for a period of time, and, as I was about to leave, she suddenly stated in a quiet but assured tone, "Now get the other book out." I read the book to her repeatedly. I paused at times to facilitate her interjections or responses if she so desired, and read on when she did not. On the fifth reading she suddenly interrupted to question the word memory. I asked if she knew what it meant, and she responded, "kind of, but I can't explain." I asked if she could give me an example of what she thought it meant. She stated, "it's like a picture, only it's in here (pointing to her head) and nobody else can see it but me. It's like your dreams, except you are awake." Lucia then went on to tell me about a dream she had where her baby brother appeared to her coming down from heaven like a tiny angel. When asked what he had said, she stated, "he didn't speak, he just stayed with me and smiled, then, when he was going back to heaven, he opened his arms out for me." I asked Lucia if she had any memories to share. She smiled shyly and nodded. Again pointing to herself she stated, "in here, it's all in here. My father and my mommy and Carlos, they are all in here now."

References

1. Department of Health and Human Services (1988). *Secretary's Work Group on Pediatric HIV Infection and Disease*. Washington, DC: Superintendent of Documents, U.S. Government Printing Office, p. 13.
2. Falloon, J., Eddy, J., Wiener, L. et al. (1989). Human immunodeficiency virus infection in children. *Journal of Pediatrics*, 114(1):10.
3. Boland, M.G., Tasker, M., Evans, P.M., et al. (1987). Helping Children with AIDS: The role of the child welfare worker. *Public Welfare* 26.
4. Garcia-Preto, N. (1982). Puerto Rican families. In McGoldrick, M., Pearce, J.K. and Giordano, J. (Eds.), *Ethnicity and Family Therapy*. New York: Guilford, p. 164.
5. Kübler-Ross, E. (1969). *On Death and Dying*. New York: Macmillan Publishing Company.

7 The Intravenous Drug User and AIDS

A. Billy S. Jones, MSW, CDAC

Bid a singer in the chorus, know thyself; and will he not turn for the knowledge to the others, his fellows in the chorus, and to his harmony with them?

—Epictetus

It is not unusual for the most sympathetic and understanding health care worker to become exasperated and judgmental when having to respond to the need of a patient or client known to be a nonrecovering (and often also noncompliant) substance abuser. Once a patient/client is identified as an addict, medical intervention is often kept to a minimum and the primary objective becomes that of quickly getting the addict out of the door or into someone else's caseload. For example,

> "Steve," an addict since the age of eight (by his recall), learned that he was HIV-positive in 1985. He survives from income obtained from male prostitution (although he does not perceive or define himself as gay or bisexual), shoplifting and selling drugs. He lives in abandoned buildings, in incarcerated settings, or with a client for short terms. Steve has been hospitalized several times a year since 1985 because of repeated bouts of opportunistic infectious diseases related to his HIV status. He is reputed to be demanding, hostile, and uncooperative with nurses, doctors, or any "authority" figure. AIDS service organizations refer him to drug treatment programs; drug treatment programs refer him to...No one has ever developed a comprehensive case management intervention to address Steve's needs as an addict and as a person with AIDS.

An even greater hostility is displayed toward the patient/client who has a dual diagnosis of HIV infection and chemical dependency. Long before health professionals were confronted with treating HIV/AIDS-related disorders in the 1980s, addicts were experiencing discrimination and humiliation in the forms of inferior or no health care, personal degradation and being declared "bad" persons, and denial of the very support systems (i.e. housing, employment, education) they needed to avoid relapse and to stay off drugs, alcohol, and other addictive substances.

> On a recent hospitalization for an HIV-related illness, Steve pointed out that he had an abscess resulting from his injecting drug use. The doctor reprimanded him for continuing to use drugs, refused to place him on methadone, and informed him that he "deserved to have AIDS since he would not stop shooting up." It was not until 24 hours later, and through the efforts of another doctor who understood that chemical addiction was a disease, that appropriate intervention for AIDS and chemical dependency was administered.

Part of the problem faced by health-care providers is that we live in a throw-away society in which we often attempt to "address" the needs of addicts by getting rid of them, by referring them to someone else, or by discharging them. Similarly, when working with those with HIV we often treat the opportunistic infection related to HIV without treating the physiologic aspects resulting from addiction.

Another problem faced by health-care providers is a lack of understanding about what chemical dependency (i.e., addiction, alcoholism, drug abuse, etc.) is and what interventions are appropriate. It is crucial that health-care workers recognize that, like HIV infection, addiction requires a holistic medical intervention that addresses the physical, psychological, and social-behavior patterns of the individual.

It is also crucial that health-care providers understand that, like persons living with AIDS/HIV infection as a chronic but manageable disease, chemical dependency is also a chronic but manageable disease. In other words, several times in a treatment program for most addicts is seldom enough for sustaining recovery. The most successful intervention model is one that is ongoing for the life span of the addict. If we stop treating the addiction, relapse may be imminent.

> "Thelma" went through seven drug treatment programs in four years. She has now been "clean and sober" for five years. She reports that *all* of the treatment programs were beneficial for her recovery since she still recalls something said or someone's story which helps her avoid relapse today. When asked which program helped her the most, she shrugs and says quite frankly, she doesn't know; she just realized that she was not a bad person, but was caught up in an unhealthy and life-threatening situation of drinking and drugging.

What Is Addiction/Chemical Dependency

Whereas there are many definitions for chemical dependency and addiction, professional associations such as the National Council of Alcoholism and the American Medical Association would agree that:

Chemical dependency is a disease characterized by the repetitive and compulsive ingestion of any psychoactive substance, in such a way as to result in interference with some aspect of the person's life; be it his/her health, family, career, or other required social adaptations and expectations for that individual.

—Stanley Gitlow, M.D.

Alcoholism/drug abuse is a chronic, progressive potentially fatal, primary disease characterized by tolerance, physical dependence, pathologic organ changes—all of which is the direct or indirect consequence of the alcohol or drug ingested.

—Vernon Johnson, Ph.D.[1]

Physiology, not psychology, determines whether a drinker or drug user will become addicted or chemically dependent. The addict's genes, enzymes, hormones, brain, and other body chemistries work together to create the individual's reaction to the chemical substance.

—James Milam, Ph.D.[2]
Katherine Ketcham

Beyond the Intravenous Drug User

Many of us have a stereotype image of who is an addict, who is an alcoholic, and who is an IV drug user. Electronic and print media have made us aware of the dysfunctional addict who is unemployed, who lives on the street, and who repeatedly injects himself with needles shared by others in a shooting gallery. However, we should be aware that the vast majority of addicts do not fit this image; in fact, many addicts are functioning addicts who may be our co-workers, neighbors, or relatives and loved ones in our homes.

"Ernest" has been employed for 12 years as an accountant with a large corporation. He is well respected by his co-workers and is often the "life of the party." Although this is known only to a select few, Ernest smokes marijuana every morning before work, during his lunch breaks, and evenings after work. He also snorts cocaine on weekends and occasionally "speedballs" cocaine and heroin by injection. Because Ernest is holding a respected position and appears to be coping with day-to-day events, very few persons acknowledge him to be a drug addict—not even his doctor.

While focus on HIV/AIDS has highlighted the fact that the sharing of drug paraphernalia (needles, syringes, cookers, water, cotton) is a major risk factor for the transmission of HIV infection, not enough stress has been placed on the HIV risk factors associated with non-injected drugs. Non-injected drugs (e.g., alcohol, crack, cocaine, poppers, ice, pills, etc.) are mood altering substances and often play a key part in users' throwing caution aside and engaging in unsafe sexual activities.

Since all drugs (including nicotine and caffeine) compromise the immune system, HIV-infected persons need to be educated that continued use of drugs may be a cofactor that may cause the progression of HIV infection to an opportunistic infection or full-blown, frank AIDS. Thus, intervention targeting known addicts as well as the general population must not only address issues relevant to "intravenous" drug users, but also those relating to the substance abusers who may not be injecting and may not be perceived as addicts.

In today's era of newer and more powerful drugs continually being introduced in the subcultures of drug abusers, most addicts are polydrug users—for example, cocaine and heroin (known as speedball), alcohol and Valium, phencyclidine (PCP) and crack. While addicts usually have a preference for one drug over another, it is common practice to combine drugs for the purpose of avoiding getting too high (an "upper") or too low (a "downer"), to go higher (e.g., marijuana laced with PCP), or to compensate for the absence of a drug at a time of craving or feeling ill (alcohol in lieu of heroin).

> Steve's drug of choice is heroin. However, when he cannot get together enough money to purchase heroin, he will drink alcohol.
>
> Ernest's drug of choice is cocaine. But on workdays he settles for smoking marijuana.
>
> Thelma's drug of choice is alcohol. She was also using tranquilizers prescribed by her doctor for depression.

Many addicts who try to stop using their drug of choice or an illegal drug may switch to a more socially acceptable drug (such as beer or wine). Health-care providers can play a key role in helping addicts understand that the ultimate goal for a recovering addict is abstinence. Even the recovering heroin addict who opts for methadone maintenance or intervention should strive for abstinence as part of his long term treatment plan.

Some narcotic medications prescribed for the treatment of an opportunistic infection related to AIDS or pain experienced by the PWA may trigger addiction for the first time or may trigger a relapse for the PWA who has been drug free for years. In fact, some recovering addicts may refuse certain medical interventions because of the fear that their addiction may be triggered. Counseling and sensitivity on the part of medical service providers is crucial for the recovering PWA to be able to make key decisions regarding his life.

> Thelma initially refused to take AZT or any medication prescribed by her doctor because she was fearful that the drugs being prescribed were addictive narcotics. Her doctor had initially failed to take her recovery into considera-tion and was interpreting her refusal to take AZT as being "uncooperative" and giving in to the disease of HIV. After some sensitive education (for the doctor and Thelma), and assurances that Thelma could be empowered to take part in her treatment plan, a holistic intervention plan was put in place. Thelma now understands that AZT is not an addictive narcotic drug and has contracted with her doctor at what point she—not he—will be willing for her to take AZT.

Many ethical issues may be raised regarding appropriate medical treatment and intervention for the PWA/HIV-positive person with a history of addiction: needle exchange programs and distribution of bleach for sterilization of drug paraphernalia, priority to appropriate drug treatment programs for addicts known to be HIV-positive, willingness of hospitals to provide quality treatment to PWA addicts with or without insurance coverage, accessibility of drug protocol clinical trails and how such access may impact not only the PWA's immune system but also his addiction, access to methadone maintenance programs and questioning the possibility that methadone may be a cofactor for the progression of HIV to full-blown AIDS—keeping in mind that *all* drugs compromise the immune system. Therefore, what is the appropriate medical intervention for the PWA addict who is still using street drugs? What is the impact of HIV prophylactic drugs (i.e. AZT, dideooxyinosine (DDI), aerosol pentamidine) on the PWA addict who continues to use illicit drugs or socially acceptable drugs such as alcohol, nicotine, or caffeine?

There are no easy answers to any of these questions, but health- care providers must be mindful of these issues and raise them with all persons involved in the treatment and intervention of the PWA/HIV-positive addict. Whatever the beliefs and desires of health-care providers may be, ultimately the PWA must be the one to make the decision about his treatment.

Treatment Intervention in Diverse Settings

Addicts go through a number of agencies and programs that may prove to be ideal settings for HIV education, emotional support, and medical treatment. The health-care provider has to keep in mind that the patient/client has at least a dual medical diagnosis—that of addiction and that of HIV infection. Until the individual's addiction has been addressed (or at least until the person is detoxified), health-care workers will have limited success with interventions attempting to treat opportunistic infections or to provide emotional and community support for the addict.

Treatment modalities for addicts are social and medical detoxification programs which may last anywhere from 48 hours to 28 days; outpatient methadone maintenance programs which may be several months or several years in duration; short-term residential and outpatient programs which may be up to ninety days in length; and long-term residential programs which may be 3 to 24 months in duration (most being 6 to 12 monthly long). Unfortunately, the amount of insurance coverage an individual has is often a determining factor of how long an individual can remain in a program. However, the vast majority of addicts in need of treatment programs do not have insurance or other financial means of paying for services. The impact of this "catch-22" dilemma is that in many cities there are often long waiting lists of persons seeking to get into publicly funded programs and empty beds at private treatment programs.

Since Steve has no fixed place of residence, carries no identification, and has no legal means of income, it is difficult for him to get into the city's methadone maintenance program which has a three-month waiting list. As an addict, Steve is often too dysfunctional to follow through with appointments and service providers are not able to break through the red tape to get him treatment on demand.

When Ernest's supervisor recognized that Ernest had a drug "problem," a treatment slot was immediately found and the company insurance policy covered all of the expenses.

As an alcoholic, Thelma was able to get into a medical detoxification unit but not into a residential treatment program. Therefore, she continued to relapse until she surrendered to the 12-step program of Alcoholics Anonymous by attending 90 meetings in 90 days. Eventually, a residential slot opened and Thelma was able to take advantage of a structured program.

One's HIV antibody status should never be a reason for denying an addict access to treatment. All employees in chemical dependency programs should be aware of and follow universal health precautions and the guidelines recommended for health care professionals by the CDC[3] and the American Medical Society on Alcoholism and Other Drug Dependence (AMSAODD).[4] All addicts should be able to access quality treatment for addiction, HIV infection, and any other medical services deemed necessary by assessments.

Intervention treatment models vary from program to program and depend in part on the philosophy of the program and staff, the primary substance the addict may be in recovery for, the duration of the program, and the training and skills for staff. Seldom do addicts make a full recovery based on one treatment intervention; in fact, most addicts who finally succeed at staying "clean and sober" have several relapses and go through several different treatment programs over a period of several years. We have come to understand that, like HIV infection, recovery from addiction is a life-long intervention. The addict has to always work on a program of intervention to avoid relapse or slips and to stay healthy.

In assessing the usefulness of a treatment program that one may be referring addicts to, several components should be in place as part of the intervention: detoxification under supervision, education components that teach the addict what chemical dependency is, one-on-one counseling, group counseling, family counseling (to address issues of co-dependency and enabling), nutrition education, stress reduction skills, education modules on HIV/AIDS issues, human sexuality, and communication skills, relapse prevention and intervention, aftercare and follow-up, and outside support networks such as 12-step programs (i.e., Alcoholics Anonymous, Cocaine Anonymous or Narcotic Anonymous). It is unlikely that all of these components will be a part of one program; thus, an integrated approach may be needed to assure the best intervention response based on the personal need of the addict seeking treatment.

Intervention for Addicts Not in Treatment

No treatment intervention works unless the addict is ready and willing to surrender to a program fully. Health-care workers can, and should, encourage addicts to get into treatment, but the reality is that the person may not be emotionally ready at that time or a treatment spot may not be available; thus the addict continues to drink, snort, or inject drugs and may be placing himself at risk for HIV infection by sharing drug paraphernalia or engaging in at-risk sexual activities while under the influence of mood altering substances.

Community street outreach programs have been organized across the country as a way to reach addicts who are not in treatment or recovery. Several modes of intervention are possible: 1) distributing literature and "Just Say No" drug messages as well as safer sex messages; 2) distributing one ounce vials of bleach to addicts and teaching them how to sterilize their syringes and cookers by flushing them with bleach and rinsing with water; and 3) exchanging clean needles for used needles with addicts who turn in needles. The extent of intervention depends on the drug and paraphernalia laws of the community, the attitudes toward and politics regarding drugs and AIDS, and the extent of HIV infection and substance abuse in the community. Outreach workers always attempt to make referrals not only to drug treatment programs, but also to HIV antibody test sites, venereal disease/sexually transmittal disease (VD/STD) clinics, shelters and food kitchens, and other community social service agencies. Messages about safer sex practices are also given. Most community street outreach programs hire recovering addicts, ex-offenders, and retired sex workers (prostitutes and hustlers) who have proven to be very effective at reaching and teaching addicts not in treatment.

Community street outreach workers appear to be having a great deal of success affecting the knowledge, attitude, and behavior of addicts not in treatment. Studies show that most addicts have at least a layperson's knowledge of HIV/AIDS, understand that they should not share drug equipment, and do make efforts to sterilize their works or refuse to share. The weakness of these changes being made by addicts is that they appear not to be sustained over a long period of time.

References

1. Johnson, V. (1980). *I'll Quit Tomorrow*. San Francisco: Harper & Row.
2. Milam, J. (1983). *Under the Influence*. New York: Bantam Books.
3. Centers for Disease Control (1988). Universal precautions for prevention of transmission of HIV, hepatitis B virus, and other bloodborne pathogens in health-care settings. *Morbidity and Mortality Weekly Report*, 37(24):377-382, 387-388.
4. American Medical Society on Alcoholism and Other Drug Dependencies (1987). *Guidelines for Facilities Treating Chemically Dependent Patients at Risk for AIDS or Infected by HIV*. Miami, FL: AMSAODD.

PART TWO

The Professional Perspective

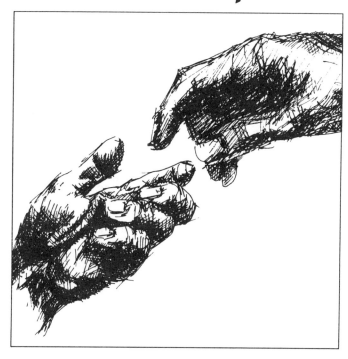

See me, feel me, touch me, heal me.

—From *Tommy*

8 The Medical Aspects of AIDS

Arnaldo Gonzales-Aviles, MD

It is a modern plague: The first great pandemic of the second half of the 20th century

—Robert C. Gallo[1]

Introduction

Three descriptive terms are used to characterize a disorder that has evolved in recent years—the acquired immunodeficiency syndrome (AIDS). The definitions of these terms are simple: *acquired immunodeficiency* means a non-genetic condition produced by influences originating outside the organism with the final result of a deficiency in the immune response; a *syndrome* is defined as a set of symptoms that occur together; a *symptom complex* is the sum of signs of any morbid state.[2] The first description of AIDS in the medical literature occurred in June 1981, in the CDC *Morbidity and Mortality Weekly Report* (MMWR) which described findings of PCP and Kaposi's sarcoma in young homosexual men.[3] Both illnesses were extremely rare in such a population. Eventually it was shown that these illnesses resulted from a deficient immunologic system, and the signs and symptoms formed a complex disorder, which was labeled AIDS.

The spread of AIDS is worldwide. Chin and Mann[4] describe three distinct patterns of infection throughout the globe. These are based on predominant risk behaviors for HIV transmission.[4] The first type is seen mostly in North America, Western Europe, Australia, New Zealand and parts of Latin America. Cases are mostly seen in homosexuals and intravenous drug abusers (IVDA), while heterosexual transmission is small, but increasing. Transmission by contaminated blood occurred in the late 1970s through 1985. Transfusion cases have since been reduced due to screening of potential donors and testing of blood and blood products. Male/female ratio ranges from 10:1 to 15:1, and population seroprevalence is anywhere from less than 1 percent to 50 percent, depending on the groups tested.

The second pattern involves southern, central and eastern Africa, as well as some Latin American countries. Spread is mostly heterosexual although trans-

Table 8-1

Distribution of AIDS per State: February 28, 1991

New York	35,823
California	31,566
Florida	14,847
Texas	11,901
New Jersey	10,753
Illinois	4,938
Puerto Rico	5,305
Pennsylvania	4,586
Massachusetts	3,150

Statistics are from the *CDC Monthly Surveillance Report.*[5]

mission through blood transfusions is common. Population seroprevalence rates are between 1 and 20 percent in sexually active people in urban areas. Eastern Europe, North Africa, the Middle East, Asia and most of the Pacific (excluding Australia and New Zealand) compromise the third group. In these areas a small number of cases have been reported.

The United States falls into the first pattern. The Public Health Service predicts that the number of infected individuals with the causative agent of AIDS is between 945,000 and 1,400,000.[5] The total number of AIDS patients in the United States as of February 28, 1991 was 167,803 of which 164,900 were adults and 2,903 were children.[5] More than 50 percent in each category are now dead. The distribution across the nation is uneven (Table 8-1). The five major states affected are New York, California, Florida, Texas and New Jersey.

Since 1981, science has studied this malady and significant progress has been made. We know much about its etiology, transmission, manifestations, statistics, methods of prevention and other important aspects, but we still lack a cure. This chapter presents a review of the current facts of this syndrome with the understanding that everyday information is obtained and further sources must be available to upgrade ourselves in this crisis.

Etiology of Aids

From observations of the initial populations effected by AIDS, several theories over why these patients were immunosuppressed developed. The major groups affected then were, homosexual men, IVDAs and hemophiliacs. All had a decrease in a specific cell of the immune system, the T-helper cell. Many in the scientific community considered the possibility of an infectious organism causing AIDS. The major organisms suspected were CMV, which was already associated with immunosuppression in kidney transplant patients; Epstein-Barr virus, an organism known to be lymphotropic; and hepatitis B, a virus of high incidence in these groups. Although these organisms were possible causative agents, they could not account for the symptoms that were currently manifested. Various laboratories independently postulated another entity, a member of the retrovirus family. Dr. Robert Gallo and his colleagues had discovered the human T-lymphotropic retrovirus (HTLV I and HTLV II) to be the causative agent of T-cell leukemia and lymphoma. Dr. Gallo and others believed that this virus or a related one was the cause of this new illness, as it also infected the T-helper cell, was transmitted sexually and/or intravenously, and was similar to the feline leukemia T-lymphotropic retrovirus that caused immunosuppression and leukemia in cats. Studies in AIDS patients showed that in a third of the cases, there were antibodies cross-reacting with HTLV. In 1984 the virus was isolated and named HTLV III, and was later renamed human immunodeficiency virus (HIV). The origin of the virus is believed to be Africa, and genetic studies demonstrate that it may have evolved 50 to 100 years ago.[6] Evidence indicates that the first probable case of AIDS occurred in 1952, and the first serum sample positive for HIV was found in 1959 in Zaire in Central Africa.[7,8]

Human Immunodeficiency Virus

HIV is a member of the Retroviridae family. This family is a member of the ribonucleic acid (RNA) viruses, which are covered by a lipid envelope, and which measure approximately 80 to 130 nm. The name "retrovirus" comes from their replicating method. In their structure is an enzyme, *reverse transcriptase*, which has the capacity to produce viral deoxyribonucleic acid (DNA) from the host DNA by using a template of its viral RNA. The reverse order in DNA production by this enzyme is what identifies this family.[9]

The Retroviridiae are subclassified into three groups or families: Lentivirinae, of which HIV is an example and which are associated with a prolonged latency between infection and evidence of the illness; Spumavirinae, which are known to produce foamy vacuolation of infected cells in cultures but are not known to produce any illnesses; and Oncovirinae, which are known to produce tumors. HTLV-1 is an example of an oncovirus.[9,10]

The structure of HIV consists externally of a membrane or envelope in an icosahedral sphere pattern with 72 spikes of glycoproteins (GPs) (GP120 and GP41). Internally is another coat of proteins, a core (p24) which contains the viral RNA and the enzyme, reverse transcriptase (Figure 8-1). The life cycle of the virus starts by entering a host. The GP120 area of the virus then binds to the surface of a host cell on a specific area called CD4. Cell fusion then occurs. Once in the cell the cytoplasm uncovers the envelope. The reverse transcriptase then proceeds to produce viral DNA from the host's DNA. This provirus then enters the cell nucleus of the host and integrates into a host chromosome to produce more viral proteins and therefore more HIVs. Once integrated into the human DNA, the virus may lay dormant for an indeterminate period of time. On activation of the infected cell, a total of eight different proteins are produced. The formed viral RNA unites with other viral proteins and buds out through the host's cellular membrane taking some GPs and forming its typical membrane.

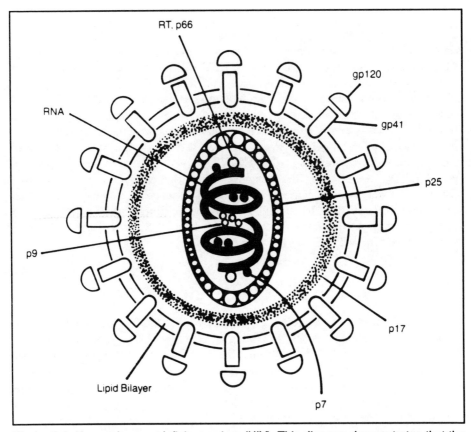

Figure 8-1. Human Immunodeficiency virus (HIV). This diagram demonstrates that the virus is composed of several spheres, each of which contain specific proteins. The outer envelope contains GP120 which attaches to T cells. The inner side of the core capsule is covered by p17, while the nucleoid contains p7 and p9. RT = reverse transcriptase. *Adapted from Tailcuff, H.I. In Levy, J.A. (1989). Human immunodeficiency virus and the pathogenesis of AIDS. Journal of the American Medical Association, 251(20):2999. Used with permission.*

The host cell is killed and the new viruses proceed to infect other cells and continue to replicate.[10]

HIV tends to have a predilection for infecting the T-cell (CD-4 positive) lymphocyte, and as a result, a major feature of this illness is a gradual decrease in these lymphocytes. This cell plays a central role in the body's immune response to an antigen or infection, leaving the individual defenseless against infections and malignancies. Although cells may also be infected, CD4 seems to be the most common site of infection.[9]

HIV Infection

Although several classifications exist for the description of HIV infection, perhaps the most widely used is from the CDC which has divided the different manifestations of infection in four clinical stages. Stage I, or the acute infection, begins the moment the individual is infected. Case reports have demonstrated the existence of a "flu-like syndrome" at this stage. Characteristics of this phase are fevers, rash (in a roseola-like pattern), pain in the joints (or arthralgia), lymphadenopathy, and rarely, neurologic syndromes, such as aseptic meningitis, acute encephalitis, myelopathy and neuropathies. This collection of symptoms is usually followed by seroconversion within 1 to 12 weeks after exposure.[13] At this point the individual enters into a chronic phase, as seen in stages II-IV.[11] The period of time to develop the end point is unknown. Research has attempted to identify precipitating or accelerating factors to the final state. Recreational drug use was once thought to advance these stages at a faster rate, however, work by Kaslow et al. has shown no statistical difference in progression rate of the illness in HIV-positive substance abusers versus HIV-positive non-substance abusers.[12] Among other factors thought to accelerate the progression of the disease is the possibility of multiple concomitant viral infections, such as herpes zoster and others.

Stage II is called the asymptomatic phase. In this stage individuals are HIV-positive but have no manifestations of the illness. It is at this stage that the virus is most likely incorporated into the DNA of the host.[11]

Stage III is known as persistent generalized lymphadenopathy. Here enlarged lymph nodes are evident, mostly affecting the inguinal, submandibular and axillary nodes. Biopsy may be required at this point, as other illnesses such as Hodgkin's disease or other infections may show similar signs and symptoms. It is important to know that not all individuals go through each phase or in the same order.[11]

The final phase is Stage IV. Eventually a high percentage of individuals infected with HIV reach this phase. Some studies show that individuals have a 40 percent chance to reach this stage in seven years once they are HIV-positive.[13] This phase results from a decrease in the immune system, particularly the T-helper cell (or CD4+). Constitutional symptoms may appear; these are debilitation, diarrhea, night sweats and fever. All of these symptoms together are known as the AIDS-related complex (ARC), although patients may demonstrate other symptoms indicative of AIDS. Examples of these are neurologic diseases such as dementias, myelopathies and peripheral neuropathies; infections; secondary cancers; or other conditions.[11] We will review below some of the manifestations of the impaired immune system. Let us start on the surface of the body.

Skin. Perhaps the most disturbing area of manifestation to individuals is that of the skin. The skin areas most frequently affected are those areas exposed to the sun such as the face, neck and trunk. Some manifestations such as Kaposi's sarcoma (KS) can be disfiguring, and as a result, patients tend to isolate themselves out of the fear of recognition of their disease by others. In general, lesions of different types are seen. We may see infections caused by parasites, fungus, viruses and bacteria; or other manifestations, including cancers such as KS, which tend to have a higher prevalence in the gay population.

Looking first at infections, of all the organisms, parasites are probably the least likely to affect the skin. Most commonly seen is scabies (*sarcoptes scabiei*).

Fungal infections are more common. The most frequently seen is *Candida albicans*, which predominantly affects oral mucosa and the esophagus. This infection can also be one of the manifestations of ARC.[11] On occasion it may infect the external skin, particularly the genital areas. Women and children (diaper rash) seem to have a higher incidence of *Candida albicans* infection than men. Another common fungal infection is from the genus Pityrosporum which causes tinea versicolor or trichophyton rubrum, causing tinea cruris and other fungal infections. Rarer cases have been observed with Cryptococco, and Histoplasma. All of these may mimic other organisms and special procedures must be performed to identify the correct pathogen for treatment.[6]

Bacterial infections are also frequently seen, Staphylococcus aureus being probably the most common. It may manifest itself as impetigo of the beard, neck, intertriginous area and abscesses. Another organism is Pseudomonas, which is commonly seen in the IVDA population and can cause skin infections, as well as systemic manifestations such as fever, malaise, etc. Multiple other organisms have also been observed and present themselves as folliculitis or impetigo.[6,13]

Viral infections are probably the most difficult to diagnose and treat. Numerous organisms have been identified that cause skin problems with viral etiology. Herpes simplex presents with skin ulcers in HIV-infected individuals (see Figure 8-2) while non-HIV-infected individuals usually present with localized vesicular lesions. Herpes simplex occurs in up to 22 percent of patients with AIDS and is seen frequently in perianal areas. However, their typical presentation may be mimicked by other organisms such as Cryptococcus and it is important to culture suspicious lesions. Herpes may also manifest itself as bulbous lesions or blisters, and may be seen in the palm of the hand. Treatment for this infection is with intravenous acyclovir, and the patient usually responds within 10 days. Molluscum contagiosum is caused by a pox virus, and is easily recognized by a typical lesion, a papule on the face, neck, and genitalia. The lesion has a pearl-white color and is umbilicated in the center. Treatment is usually surgical removal, but recurrence is common. Human papilloma virus causes venereal warts and, in addition to the typical genital lesion, it may appear on the hands and feet. Varicella zoster, a virus also known as chicken pox, is manifested by generalized besicular skin eruptions. In HIV-infected individuals it may manifest itself as pneumonia, encephalitis, and other presentation. Usually chicken pox occurs in childhood and the virus remains latent in the dorsal root ganglia of the nervous system. In later life the virus reactivates itself and causes a painful vesicular eruption on the skin localized to a dermatome or a skin region. This is commonly known as shingles. It has been observed that young adults who are HIV positive and present with shingles develop stage IV of AIDS within the very near future.[13] Other viruses infecting the skin include Epstein-Barr virus (infectious mononucleosis) and cytomegalovirus.[6]

In addition to these infections there are other conditions: seborrheic dermatitis, hair changes, drug reactions, infections of the nails and malignancies. Seborrheic dermatitis is a condition that can affect up to 5 percent of the general population. It is a very common first presentation of AIDS. It has preference for

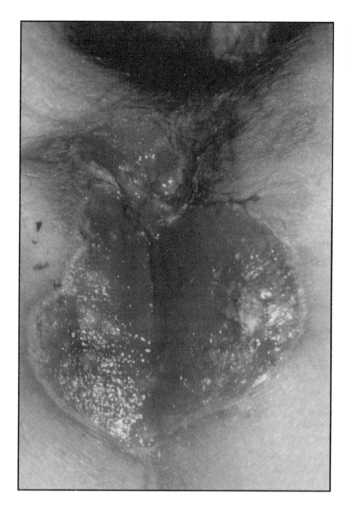

Figure 8-2. Herpes simplex affecting the perianal area.

the scalp, cheeks, trunk, groin, and extremities. Grossly there are areas of erythema with flaky desquamation and, on occasion, it may have a greasy appearance.[13]

Hair changes are common in the later stages of the illness. Reported in the literature are alopecia, frontal recession, premature graying, and in black men, loss of the natural curl in their hair. It is unclear if these findings are a direct result of the HIV infection.[13]

Nails may also be affected by fungal infection, particularly tinea rubrum. Some patients' nails may acquire a yellow color, the clinical significance of which is unclear.[13]

Of the malignancies, the most common is KS. This malignancy was first described in 1872 by Moritz Kaposi. It was a rare tumor of the skin seen mostly in Europe and North America in men over 50 years of age, of Italian Mediterranean or Eastern European Jewish ancestry. This type of KS is what is known today as classic KS. This malignancy was also seen in renal transplant patients, young adult black African males, and other patients receiving immunosuppressive therapy. The development

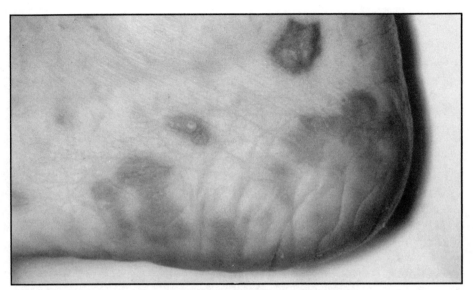

Figure 8-3. Kaposi's sacroma affecting the lateral aspect of the foot.

of KS in young gay men associated with HIV infection is known as epidemic KS (Figure 8-3). Eighteen percent of all patients initially diagnosed with AIDS present with KS. Histologically these cases are similar, but clinical manifestations and the course of the disease are different. Of all the groups at risk for HIV disease, homosexual men have the highest incidence of presentation with KS. Once a diagnosis is made, medical survival is 18 to 24 months. In AIDS the skin is most commonly affected by KS, however, the gastrointestinal, pulmonary and cardiac systems may also be affected. There are three stages in the development of KS: 1) a patch stage in which pink or red macules develop; 2) a plaque stage in which the lesions are raised and violaceous plaques or nodules develop; 3) a nodular stage in which lesions can progress to coalesce and convert into elevated nodules. Treatment depends on the location and size of the lesion. For small topical lesions, radiation therapy or surgical ablation can be used. Agents such as liquid nitrogen, dinitrochlorobenzene, or direct injections of vinblastine have been used with success. These medications act by causing a local inflammation which destroys the KS. For gastrointestinal and systemic lesions, other agents such as vinblastine, vincristine or adriamycin are used. The major problem with these agents are the side effects, which include immunosuppression and therefore the risk of depleting the immune system even further. Other agents include alpha interferon, which has shown good response.[6]

Recent reports have also shown an increase in the incidence of squamous cell carcinoma in HIV-positive individuals. The significance of this finding is unclear and requires further research.[5]

Lungs. In the respiratory system there are a variety of possible manifestations of HIV infection, which include pneumonia, malignancies, and diffuse alveolar damage.[13]

Several etiologies can cause infection of the lungs and subsequent respiratory failure. Perhaps the two most common pathogens are *Pneumocystis carinii* (PCP) and cytomegalovirus (CMV).[13] Bacterial organisms, however, are a frequent cause of pneumonias, and they usually affect HIV- infected individuals with more frequency and severity than they do the general population. The most common bacterial organisms affecting AIDS patients are *Streptococcus pneumoniae* and *Haemophillus influenzae*.[13] The clinical presentation is usually of an acute onset of symptoms which includes fevers, chills, pleuritic chest pain and a productive purulent cough. Treatment is with well-known conventional therapies.

In AIDS most pneumonias are caused by *Pneumocystis carinii*—an organism which for years was thought to be a parasite but now it is thought to be a fungus.[14] Typical features of this pneumonia are recent difficulty breathing, dry cough, mucoid sputum, inability to take a deep breath, and hypoxemia as measured by arterial gases. A chest x-ray examination may be normal and diagnosis relies on a positive sputum examination and/or bronchoscopy, where either a biopsy or a sample of bronchoalveolar washings is taken and demonstrates the organism. Two modalities of treatment exist: pentamidine isethionate given intravenously, and intravenous or oral trimetropim-sulfamethoxazole. For the first three to four days patients may not show significant improvement, and may actually deteriorate. On occasion no improvement is seen in the first 10 days. Survival rates are around 80 to 90 percent in the first episode, depending on the patient's immune status, the presence of other medical problems, the severity of pulmonary dysfunction, and tolerance to treatment. Major problems with treatment are the side effects of these medications. As many as 70 to 100 of patients on either drug experience some type of side effect. Pentamidine is associated with decreasing neutrophile counts, hyper- or hypoglycemia, hypotension, or pancreatitis. Trimetropin-sulfamethoxazole may cause skin rashes, fevers, leukopenia, hepatitis, nausea and kidney inflammations. AZT has been shown to decrease the frequency and severity of PCP episodes, while aerosol pentamidine or dapsone (medications used in the treatment of leprosy) can also decrease the number of episodes of PCP.[6,13]

Other causes of pneumonia are the viruses, which are the most difficult to diagnose and treat. Results of cultures are time consuming, and treatments are rare. CMV is probably a frequent cause of respiratory failure in these patients. This organism is also known to cause retinitis which may cause blindness. Treatment for this infection is with Ganciclovir (DHPG). This medication must be given for life and administered intravenously.[6,13]

Another frequent pulmonary manifestation is tuberculosis. This infection seems to occur more commonly in IVDAs. Treatment for it is well known and traditional.

Malignancies such as KS and other lymphomas can also occur in the lungs. Kaposi's sarcoma is known to produce massive intrapulmonary hemorrhage, which tends to be fatal. Treatment is limited due to the side effect of immunosuppression of these medications.[13]

The term "diffuse alveolar damage" has been recognized in the past in immunocompromised patients. It occurs as a result of the lungs response to injury from infections, but no causative organism has been identified.[13]

Gastrointestinal System. The gastrointestinal manifestations of AIDS are common and very disturbing to those infected. Illnesses in this area occur as a direct result of three possible sources: direct HIV infection, opportunistic infections, malignancies, or any combination of these three.[11]

Difficulty swallowing, with or without retrosternal pain, is one of the most common symptoms seen. One of the causative organisms is *Candida albicans*, a fungal infection that produces oral thrush. This gives the tongue and oral mucosa a thick white layer with cheese-like appearance. If it infects the esophagus it may produce dysphagia and retrosternal pain. Additionally it may infect other areas such as the stomach, and it may disseminate; however, it is rare to see this complication in HIV infection. Treatment is with anesthetics and antifungal medication.[6] Other organisms causing esophagitis include viruses such as herpes simplex virus (herpes virus huminis). This organism can also affect the mouth and perianal areas. It does not cause diarrhea, as it usually invades the final segments of the gut. Common signs and symptoms are dysphagia and retrosternal pain, anorectal pain with constipation or obstipation, and the presence of small coalescent vesicles with raised friable borders.[6] In patients with weight loss, diarrhea and malabsorption, CMV may be a causative agent. Of the bacteria, Salmonella can frequently affect the gastrointestinal (GI) system, producing fever and shaking chills. This organism frequently is the cause of bacteremia in AIDS.[6,13]

Another major manifestation in this system is hepatitis which may be caused by CMV, mycobacteria, cryptosporidium, Cryptococcus, or frequently by drugs. On occasion this condition requires discontinuation of all treatments, for the liver can tolerate a limited amount of insult, and most drugs are metabolized by the liver.[13]

Finally, there is HIV wasting syndrome. This condition most likely occurs as a result of the direct HIV infection on the gastrointestinal tract.

> HIV wasting syndrome is defined by the CDC as findings of profound involuntary weight loss plus either chronic diarrhea (at least two loose stools per day for more than 30 days) or chronic weakness and documented fever (for more than 30 days, intermittent or constant) in the absence of a concurrent illness or condition other than HIV infection that could explain the findings.[15]

The cause of this presentation is unclear; studies have demonstrated the virus in epithelium of the bowels, in particular the neuroendocrine cells. This condition probably decreases the GI mobility and function, and therefore decreases the ability to digest and absorb nutrients, thus causing the above-mentioned symptoms.[13]

Neurological System. Of the new cases expected by 1992, approximately 30 to 40 percent will have nervous system involvement.[16] Again, the manifestations of symptoms in this area will be seen either as a direct effect of the HIV infection or as a result of opportunistic infections (parasites, fungi, viruses and bacteria) and/or other malignancies of the nervous system. The most common infection is probably caused by the parasite *Toxoplasma gondii*. This organism can cause a severe necrotizing encephalitis and/or vasculitis.[17] This condition occurs in 5 to 15 percent of patients, who present with lethargy, confusion, focal neurologic signs, altered level of consciousness and seizures. In autopsy cases it has been found in 10 to 30 percent of patients depending on the group and population studied.[18] Diagnosis can be done with structural brain imaging techniques such as computed tomography (CT scan) and/or magnetic resonance imaging (MRI), however, it is often difficult to differentiate from cancers. Most centers recommend a treatment trial prior to invasive diagnostic tests to reach a diagnosis. Treatment of this infection is with sulfadiazines and pyrimethamine indefinitely, since discontinuation may cause recurrence.[11]

Fungal infections are caused by Cryptococcus, Histoplasma, Candida, Aspergillus, and others. Of these, the most frequent infection is by *cryptococcus neoformans*. It usually causes meningitis or a parenchymal lesion of the brain.[13] Clinical presentation is with headaches, nausea, vomiting, confusion, and lethargy. For diagnosis a spinal fluid analysis is required. Treatment consists of IV amphotericin (other medications are currently in active research) for life.

Viral agents are very difficult to diagnose in a patient with neurologic manifestations. The most common agents are papova, CMV and herpes simplex. CMV is often confused with HIV encephalopathy, but essentially affects the grey matter of the brain, while HIV affects subcortical areas. It may also infect the spinal cord, causing myelopathy and radiculopathy. CMV is very difficult to diagnose when even spinal fluid cultures have been negative. However, if CMV is suspected, treatment should be initiated. Progressive multifocal leukoencephalitis is a neurologic condition caused by the human papovavirus JC. This organism has a predilection for infecting a specific cell in the nervous system, the oligodendrocyte.[19] In this condition there is a selective demyelinization of nerves; clinical evolution is slow and focal neurologic signs such as hemiplegia and paralysis have been observed. There is no treatment for this condition, and usually it is lethal; however, sporadic cases of successful treatment have been reported.[13]

Bacterial agents include neurosyphilis, *Escherichia coli*, MAI and *mycobacterium tuberculosis*. This last organism is most commonly seen in the IVDA population, and may require brain biopsy for proper diagnosis.[11]

Neoplasms of the brain have been reported in up to five percent of autopsy findings. Lymphomas (usually B-cell type) occur in up to one to two percent of all AIDS patients. These patients present with generalized lethargy, confusion and seizures. The most common areas affected are the cerebrum, cerebellum and less often the brain stem. On CT or MRI multiple white lesions are evident. Kaposi's sarcoma is another malignancy reported, but it is very rare and usually metastatic.[20]

Perhaps the most devastating presentation of HIV is its direct infection of the brain. It is known that HIV passes the blood-brain barrier and enters the central nervous system at a very early phase of the illness.[21] In addition to its direct effect on the brain, it infects the spinal cord, the peripheral nervous system and skeletal muscles. Different terms have been used to describe the clinical presentation of its infection on the brain. The CDC uses the term "HIV encephalopathy"; other names in the literature include AIDS dementia complex (ADC), subacute encephalitis and AIDS encephalopathy.

> HIV encephalopathy is defined as clinical findings of disabling cognitive and/or motor dysfunction interfering with occupation or activities of daily living, or loss of behavioral developmental milestones affecting a child, progressing over weeks to months, in the absence of a concurrent illness or condition other than HIV infection that could explain the findings. Methods to rule out such concurrent illnesses and conditions must include cerebrospinal fluid examination and either brain imaging (computed tomography, or magnetic resonance) or autopsy.[15]

Clinically, there are a variety of presentations, but in general there is a decline in any of three major areas: cognitive, motor and behavioral.

Direct HIV infection has been found in up to 25 to 40 percent of autopsy cases.[18] The mechanism of action for its presentation is unclear. A theory involves the GP120 molecule of the external capsule of the virus. It is known that the chemical structure of this protein is similar to a nerve trophic (nutritional) factor called neuroleukin. Researchers believe that GP120 blocks this trophic factor and as a result the nerve dies.[22] Treatment of HIV encephalopathy with AZT has been effective in some cases.

Conclusion

AIDS is an illness caused by HIV. There is currently no cure for the disease, however, pharmacotherapy exists to delay the progression of HIV infection. An example of this is Zidovidine (azidothymidine) [AZT], a drug that in clinical trials proved to delay disease progression in HIV-infected patients with a CD4 lymphocyte count of less than 500 cells/mm.[23] Vaccines and other drugs are currently being investigated for the prevention and delay of progression to AIDS. The availability of these drugs should be an incentive for HIV testing of all individuals at risk, in view that if tests results are positive, there is treatment to avoid developing stages III and IV. With respect to prevention, in lieu of the possible availability of a vaccine in the future, a major preventive method available to all is education. To prevent HIV infection, everyone must avoid risky sexual behavior, or sharing drug needles and syringes.

This chapter has briefly summarized the enormous progress and findings on AIDS in the last ten years. The importance of updating oneself with recent AIDS literature cannot be emphasized enough, as education and therefore prevention of infection is perhaps the single best weapon against this disease.

References

1. Gallo, R.C. (1987). The AIDS virus. *Scientific American*, 256(1) (January):47.

2. Hensyl, W.R. (Ed.) (1982). *Illustrated Stedman's Medical Dictionary*, 24th ed. Baltimore: Williams & Wilkins.

3. Friedman-Kien, A., Laubenstein, L. Marmoor, M., et al (1981). KS and PCP among homosexual men—New York City and California. *Morbidity and Mortality Weekly Report*, 30: 305-308.

4. Chin, J. and Mann, J.M. (1988). The global patterns and prevalence of AIDS and HIV infection. *AIDS* 2(Suppl 1): S247-S252.

5. Centers for Disease Control. *AIDS Monthly Surveillance Report*, March.

6. DeVita, V.T., Hellman, S. and Rosenberg, S.A. (1988). *AIDS Etiology, Diagnosis, Treatment and Prevention*, 2nd ed. Philadelphia: J.B. Lippincott.

7. Huminer, D., Rosenfeld, J.B. and Pitlik, S.D. (1987). AIDS in the pre-AIDS era. *Reviews of Infectious Diseases*, 9:1102-1108.

8. Nahmas, A.J., Weiss, J., Yao, X., et al. (1986). Evidence for human infection with an HTLV III/LAV-like virus in Central Africa 1959 (letter). *Lancet*, i:1279-1280.

9. Ho, D.D., Pomerantz, R.J. and Kaplan, J.C. (1987). Pathogenesis of infection with human immunodeficiency virus. *The New England Journal of Medicine*, 317(5):278-286.

10. Levy, J. (1989). Human immunodeficiency viruses and the pathogenesis of AIDS. *JAMA* 261(20):2997-3006.

11. Williams, I., Mindel, A. and Weller, I.V.D. (1989). *AIDS*. Philadelphia: J.B. Lippincott.

12. Kaslow, R.A., Blackwelder, W.C., Ostrow, D.G., et al. (1989). No evidence for a role of alcohol or other psychoactive drugs in accelerating immunodeficiency in HIV-1-positive individuals. *JAMA*, 261(23):3424-3429.

13. Harawi, S.J. and O'Hara, C.J. (1989). *Pathology and Pathophysiology of AIDS and HIV-Related Diseases*. St. Louis: C.V. Mosby.

14. Haque, A., Plattner, S.B., Cook, R.T., et al. (1987). PC taxonomy as viewed by electron microscopy. *American Journal of Clinical Pathology*, 87:504-510.

15. Centers for Disease Control (1987). Revision of the CDC surveillance case definition for acquired immunodeficiency syndrome. *Morbidity and Mortality Weekly Report*, 36(15) (August 14): 1s-15s.

16. Levy, R.M., Bredesen, D.E. and Rosenblaum, M.L. (1985). Neurologic manifestations of the acquired immunodeficiency syndrome (AIDS): Experience at UCSF and review of the literature. *Journal of Neurosurgery*, 62:475-495.

17. Navia, B.A., Petito, C.K., Gold, J.W. et al. (1986). Cerebral toxoplasmosis complicating the acquired immunodeficiency syndrome: Clinical and neuropathological findings in 27 patients. *Annuals of Neurology*, 19:224-238.

18. Gray, F., Gherardi, R., Baudrimont, M., et al. (1987). Leucoencephalopathy with multinucleated giant cells containing human immune deficiency virus-like particles and multiple opportunistic cerebral infections in one patient with AIDS. *Acta Neuropathology*, 73:99-104.

19. Blum, L.W., Chambers, R.A., Schwartzman, R.J., et al. (1985). Progressive multifocal leukoencephalopathy in acquired immune deficiency syndrome. *Archives of Neurology*, 42:137-139.

20. So, Y.T., Beckstead, J.H. and Davis, R.L. (1986). Primary CNS lymphoma in acquired immune deficiency syndrome. *Annuals of Neurology*, 20:566-5572.

21. Bridge, P.T., Mirsky, A.F. and Goodwin, F.K. (Eds.). (1988). *Psychological, Neuropsychiatric, and Substance Abuse Aspects of AIDS*. New York: Raven Press.

22. Lee, M.R., Ho, D.D. and Gurney, M.E. (1987). Functional interaction and partial homology between human immunodeficiency virus and neuroleukin. *Science*, 237:1047-1051.

23. Baldwin, E. (Ed.) (1990). *NIAID AIDS Agenda*. Bethesda, MD: Office of Communications, National Institute of Allergies and Infectious Diseases, March.

9 General Systems Theory
A Pragmatic View

Kent N. Tigges, MS, OTR, FAOTA, FHIH

When you look upon me, please look beyond my diseased and broken body. Please look into my eyes and see me as the person I am—frightened, scared and fighting for my life. Please guide me carefully, gently and with dignity to my life's end.

—Anonymous

Introduction

General systems theory (GST) has been a recognized and highly valued concept of model building and problem solving since the early 1960s. GST has come into and out of fashion depending on the climate of the health-care industry. The use of GST in health care has been most frequently threatened by our obsession with biomedical techniques and technology and its associated reductionistic view of intervention.

Reductionism is a single-system method of study and intervention. Its focus is to reduce phenomena into units that can be examined, studied and measured, so that their relationship to other similarly reduced units can be determined. Reductionism is based on the assumption that, by studying single units of behavior, all parts can be brought together into an understanding of the whole.[1] Boulding has stated that

> The crisis in science today arises because of the increasing difficulty of such profitable talk among scientists as a whole. Specialization has out-run trade. Communication between the disciplines becomes increasingly difficult and the Republic of Learning is breaking up into isolated subcultures with only tenuous lines of communication between them. The reason for this break-up in the Republic of Learning is specialization.[1]

Hence, professionals can only talk to, and understand, similar professionals in the same subculture. Each group has its own language and interpretation of behavior that only they can understand, forming a kind of scientific Tower of Babel. Their means and methods of intervention are employed in esoteric isolation, while giving lip service to caring for the complex needs of those individuals in their care.

There are two major faults with specialization and the resulting reductionistic approach as a conclusive model of studying and treating behavior:

1. There is no substantial evidence that the strategies of studying single units (systems) can yield a complete explanation of behavior in even the most elementary living system,

2. The reductionist view is a gross oversimplification of physical and social function and behavior.[1]

In all fairness to science and the health-care professionals who advocate specialization and reductionism, the reductionist view of the human organism has, and continues to give science a useful view of human behavior. However, it must be remembered that this useful view is also an incomplete one. To not recognize and appreciate this fact is to do a great disservice to the people who entrust their lives to our care. For example, by reducing persons with AIDS to the cellular level, scientists were able to discover that AZT could effectively slow the progression of HIV. While this is unarguably a great step forward in combatting AIDS, many of the problems at the higher systems were not addressed. For example, for AZT to be effective at the systems level, it must be administered around the clock every four hours. This requires the person with AIDS and/or their caregiver to interrupt their sleep cycle to take the medication. Sleep deprivation can then affect the person level, adding to the fatigue caused by the disease and increasing the reliance of the PWA on others. At an even higher level, that of the family, the cost of the AZT (as much as $10,000 per year) might prove strenuous or even prohibitive.

As a result of the great knowledge explosion of the past four decades, it is obvious that the generalist approach, in and of itself, is no longer appropriate or feasible in dealing with the extreme complexities of the human organism. Therefore, it would be foolish for anyone to ridicule the place or importance of specialization in health care. So where do we go from here? Are we to sacrifice one extreme for the other? Is it to be the bio-medical-reductionistic approach or the generalist approach? The answer, of course, is to do neither but rather bridge effectively and efficiently the gap between the two approaches. The logical solution is to employ the GST concept of model building and problem solving.

Steps to Understanding and Implementing General Systems Theory

The first step is to examine the elements, systems, key concepts and foci of the knowledge universe map that constitute the human being (Figure 9-1). Through examining this map one cannot be less than overwhelmed at the vast complexities of humankind's encounter with life.

Elements	Systems	Key Concepts	Focus
biosphere nation	VIII Transcendental Systems	Symbolization	Ideas
society culture	VII Cultural Systems	Culturation	Organizations
subculture community family	VI Social Systems	Socialization	
"The Person" levels of conduct and experience	V Human Systems	Adaptation	Living Organisms
systems organs tissue cells	IV Open Systems		
organelles molecules	III Thermostats of Steady States Systems	Homeostasis	Things
atoms subatomic particles	II Clockworks of Mechanical Systems	Equilibrium	
gluon plasma quarks (?)	I Frameworks of Static Systems		

Figure 9-1. The Knowledge Universe Map. *Based on Boulding, K.E. (1956). General Systems Theory — The skeleton of science. Management Science, 2:197-208.*

The second step is to apply the laws of hierarchy to the knowledge universe map. Feibleman[2] has aptly defined the laws of hierarchy that clearly and definitively describe the interrelationships and interdependencies among the elements, systems, key concepts and foci. Four of these laws are as follows:

1. The complexity of the levels increases upward. The supersystem is the most complex and the last to emerge. The subsystem is the least complex and the first to emerge.

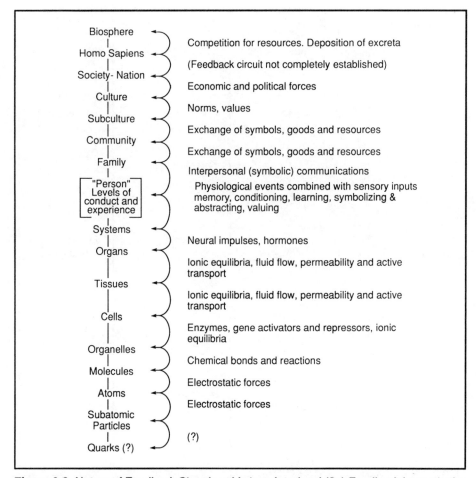

Figure 9-2. Nature of Feedback Signals at Various Interlevel (2n) Feedback Loops in the "Man" Hierarchy. *Based on Boulding, K.E. (1956). General systems theory — The skeleton of science. Management Science, 2, 197-208.*

Example: Supersystem   Family
               ↕   ↕
             System   Person
               ↕   ↕
            Subsystem   Systems
               ↕   ↕

2. The higher level (supersystem) depends upon the lower (subsystem) and the lower is directed by the higher. The supersystem is complex, the subsystem is simplistic and basic.

3. A disturbance or change in the organism at any level will affect all levels. Internal or external disturbances or changes affect all levels of the organism.

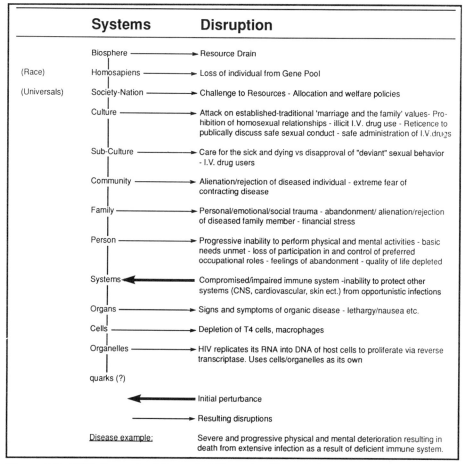

Systems   Disruption

Biosphere ⟶ Resource Drain

(Race)   Homosapiens ⟶ Loss of individual from Gene Pool

(Universals)   Society-Nation ⟶ Challenge to Resources - Allocation and welfare policies

Culture ⟶ Attack on established-traditional 'marriage and the family' values- Pro-hibition of homosexual relationships - illicit I.V. drug use - Reticence to publically discuss safe sexual conduct - safe administration of I.V. drugs

Sub-Culture ⟶ Care for the sick and dying vs disapproval of "deviant" sexual behavior - I.V. drug users

Community ⟶ Alienation/rejection of diseased individual - extreme fear of contracting disease

Family ⟶ Personal/emotional/social trauma - abandonment/ alienation/rejection of diseased family member - financial stress

Person ⟶ Progressive inability to perform physical and mental activities - basic needs unmet - loss of participation in and control of preferred occupational roles - feelings of abandonment - quality of life depleted

Systems ⟵ Compromised/impaired immune system -inability to protect other systems (CNS, cardiovascular, skin ect.) from opportunistic infections

Organs ⟶ Signs and symptoms of organic disease - lethargy/nausea etc.

Cells ⟶ Depletion of T4 cells, macrophages

Organelles ⟶ HIV replicates its RNA into DNA of host cells to proliferate via reverse transcriptase. Uses cells/organelles as its own

quarks (?)

⟵ Initial perturbance

⟶ Resulting disruptions

Disease example: Severe and progressive physical and mental deterioration resulting in death from extensive infection as a result of deficient immune system.

Figure 9-3. AIDS: Example of Spread of Disruption Through the Hierarchy. © 1989, K.N. Tigges, W.M. Marcil. Based on Boulding, K.E. (1956). General systems theory — The skeleton of science. Management Science, 2:197-208.

Stabilization between all systems must be obtained before there will be a state of homeostasis.

4. The higher level (supersystem) cannot be reduced to the lower level (subsystem). Each level has its own characteristics qualities. To ignore the qualities of the higher levels is to ignore the complexity of the organism at its lower levels.

The third step is to examine the "nature of feedback signals at various inter-level (2n) feedback loops in the 'human' hierarchy" (Figure 9-2), and again apply the laws of hierarchy.

The fourth step in the GST process is to apply the feedback signals at various inter levels (see Figure 9-2) to AIDS (Figure 9-3).

The fifth step is for each discipline represented on the interdisciplinary team to construct a conceptual model which represents their scope of practice. The occupational therapy conceptual model for palliative rehabilitation is founded on three basic assumptions and seven essential concepts. The assumptions are:

"Needs are indispensable part of human nature and imperatively demand satisfaction."[3]

"Man has need to master his environment, to alter and improve it."[3]

"There is a relationship between levels of aspiration and expectancy established in prior socialization and current patterns of success and failure."[4]

The seven concepts are motivation and locus of control, temporal adaptation, occupational roles, competence, achievement, self-esteem, and quality of life. As the understanding of the concepts of motivation and quality of life are frequently misunderstood and thus inappropriately implemented, the following definitions are given:

Motivation: "The potential for a specific behavior to occur in a given situation under circumstances where there are available reinforcements is a function of the expectancy in that situation for an available reinforcement and the value of that reinforcement in that situation."[5]

Quality of life: "Quality of life refers to the subjective satisfaction expressed of experienced by an individual in his/her physical, mental and social situation. Quality of life refers to the objective achievement by certain persons of attributes and skills that are highly valued in our culture, such as intellectual ability, physical capacity, emotional stability, artistic and technical skills, and the capacity to form and enjoy social relationships."[6] (Figure 9-4)

Each given discipline must exercise extreme caution in realistically stating their scope of practice. Paradoxically, in the quest of specialization and reductionism in the health-care system, many professionals pretend, and often sincerely believe and advocate, that they are sufficiently educated and skilled in "treating the whole person," commonly referred to as the "holistic" model of care. None of us are educated or skilled in providing holistic intervention; to think or attempt to do so is to do a great disservice to those patients under our care. Figure 9-5 identifies a variety of disciplines and their primary alignment of the primary system of their scope of practice. The sixth step is for each discipline to identify the appropriate assessment instruments and treatment strategies that are appropriate to rectify, stabilize or maintain, either temporarily or permanently, the disrupted systems.

The seventh step is an interdisciplinary task. A representative of each discipline takes their general system's generic configuration, and aligns and interfaces it with the other discipline's configuration, into a single unified systems configuration.

The eighth step is to take the unified GST configuration and compare it with the systems disease model (see Figure 9-3) to be certain there is compliance. If there is no compliance, the interdisciplinary team must examine the following issues:

1. Is a given discipline under- or over-representing their scope of practice?
2. Are there gaps in systems that need to be represented by disciplines not present on the existing interdisciplinary team?

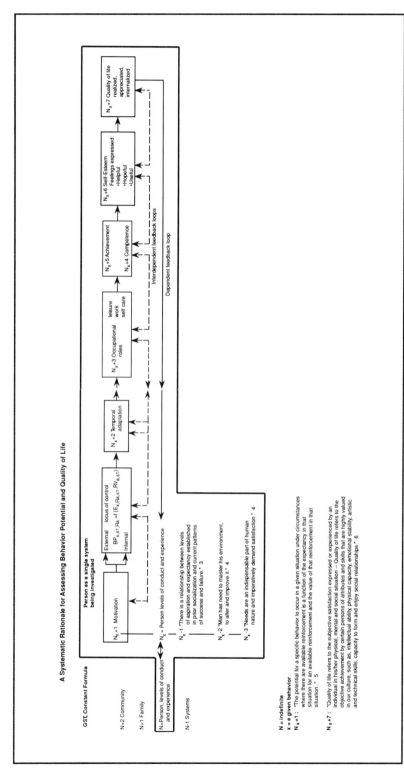

Figure 9-4. A General Systems Theory Generic Configuration of Assumptions and Concepts of Occupational Behavior: The Adult Person. © 1989, K.N. Tigges, S. Janelle.

Disciplines	Systems	Disruption
State & Federal Government }	Society-Nation	Challenge to Resources - Allocation and welfare policies
Anthropology Theology }	Culture	Attack on established-traditional 'marriage and the family' values - Prohibition of homosexual relationships - illicit I.V. drug use - Reticence to publicly discuss safe sexual conduct - safe administration of I.V. drugs
Law Local Government Epidemiology }	Sub-Culture	Care for the sick and dying vs disapproval of "deviant" sexual behavior - I.V. drug users
Psychiatry Psychology Social Work }	Family	Personal/emotional/social trauma - abandonment/alienation/rejection of diseased family member - financial stress
Occupational Therapy }	Person	Progressive inability to perform physical and mental activities - basic needs Unmet - loss of participation in and control of preferred occupational roles - feelings of abandonment - quality of life depleted
Nursing Medicine Physical Therapy }	Systems	
Immunology	Organs	Signs and symptoms of organic disease - lethargy/nausea etc.
Bio-chemistry	Cells	Depletion of T4 cells, macrophages
Virology	Organelles	HIV replicates its RNA into DNA of host cells to proliferate via reverse transcriptase. Uses cells/organelles as its own

Figure 9-5. Relationship of Interdisciplinary Input in General Systems Management. © 1989, K.N. Tigges, W.M. Marcil.

3. Can the present team appropriately, effectively and efficiently meet the complex needs of the patient? If the team decides that they cannot meet the complex needs of the patient, are they: 1) prepared to call in the necessary professionals, at least on a consulting basis, to complement the existing team? 2) content to accept that the existing/controlling agency is not prepared to pay for consultants? If so, the team must reconcile themselves to providing incomplete services. Should this be the case, the team has an ethical responsibility to convey their incomplete health-care model to the patient and his significant other(s).

The team must have consensus to proceed with an incomplete systems approach, to reconstruct their intervention plan or to seek out the appropriate disciplines that will complete the GST systems approach.

The ninth step is for the interdisciplinary team to construct collectively a patient treatment plan. It is essential that this plan be formulated as a single and unified plan. Conglomerate multi-disciplinary treatment plan construction, which occurs when each discipline designs its own individual treatment plan and melds it together into a so-called team treatment plan, is characteristic of the multi-disciplinary model of care. The major failure of this multi-disciplinary mode is that it promotes an isolationist, single-systems approach to treatment. The multi-disciplinary mode is not in compliance with GST. When the interdisciplinary team is formulating the GST treatment plan, it is paramount that the following cardinal principles be employed:

1. Regardless of the age, nature of illness, disability or impairment, be it acute or chronic, all patients are to be considered and treated as being at high risk. People's lives are very precious commodities, and must never be treated lightly, indifferently or judgmentally.
2. Each patient has the right to self-determined quality of life experiences. Therefore, the focus of assessment and intervention must attend to the following beliefs:
   a. The patient is the pivotal initiative in assessment, treatment planning, and in the determination of the expected outcomes.
   b. The patient is to be considered as a *person* first; as impaired, diseased or disabled second. The patient is are never to be considered handicapped.
   c. The patient's rights, both real and imagined, must be aligned with appropriate and realistic life responsibilities.
3. The assessment of any given patient must be reflective of, and compliant with, the discipline's general systems configuration treatment plan. Each patient has the right to specific and detailed ideographic and nomothetic attention.
4. The treatment plan must always be directly reflective of the patient's level of conduct and experiences (N = person) and the interrelationship and interdependency between the compromised subsystem (N - 1) and the super-system (N + 1).

The GST concept of model building and problem solving (understanding physical-personal-social function and behavior) may sound like a complex and time-consuming process. In reality it is not. After all, what is our mission as health-care practitioners? Are we here to serve, uncompromisingly, the complex needs of our patients, or are we here to do the least possible to meet arbitrary standards set by outside regulating agencies? To be sure, it is hoped that we can do both; always keeping first and foremost in our minds that the patient is a person and, as such, is a very precious and irreplaceable commodity in the scheme of life. People's lives, and the structure and function of the person and their family, constitute the essential stability of our society. If we do not take these factors into full and appropriate account we are not fulfilling our duty and responsibility to humanity. The general systems concept is, without question, effective, efficient and economical. Its utility is not only consumer efficient, but also payer efficient.

AIDS has poignantly illustrated that it cannot be solved from the viewpoint of studying isolated systems, just as a jigsaw puzzle cannot be assembled on the basis of a few, isolated pieces. Hopefully, AIDS will be controlled, if not eliminated, in the near future. Until such a time, we, as professionals, as well as the public at large, must recognize that the knowledge and achievements that have been accomplished thus far, although unarguably useful, are still incomplete. It is believed that if each and every one of us cooperates in a GST approach, we can appropriately and effectively solve the puzzle and riddle of AIDS. In doing so, hopefully we can bring those who collectively suffer the consequences back into the health and respect that they so rightly deserve.

References

1. Boulding, K.E. (1956). General systems theory—the skeleton of science. *Management Science*, 2:197-208.

2. Feibleman, J.K. (1954). Theory of integrated levels. *British Journal for the Philosophy of Science*, 5:59-66.

3. Reilly, M. (1962). Occupational therapy can be one of the great ideas of 20th century medicine. *American Journal of Occupational Therapy*, 16:1-9.

4. Reilly, M. (1969). The educational process. *American Journal of Occupational Therapy*, 23:299-307.

5. Rotter, J.B. (1954). *Social Learning and Clinical Psychology*. Englewood Cliffs, NJ: Prentice-Hall, pp. 197- 208.

6. Twycross, R.G. (1987). Quality before quantity: A note of caution. *Palliative Medicine*, 1(1):65-72.

10 Personal-Professional Use of Self

Kent N. Tigges, MS, OTR, FAOTA, FHIH

Death is not the ultimate tragedy of life. The ultimate tragedy is depersonalization—dying in an alien and sterile area, separated from the spiritual nourishment that comes from being able to reach out to a loving hand, separated from a desire to experience the things that make life worth living, separated from hope.[1]

N. Cousins, *Anatomy of an Illness*

Introduction

As with any other disease[2] or disability, the PWA must come to grips with, or at least achieve a measure of resolution as to how he is going to "accept" his disease, the manner in which he contracted it, and perhaps even more importantly, how he is going to deal, respond, and/or react to the feelings, attitudes or reactions of others, if he is going to appreciate even a measure of quality of life in his remaining weeks, months, or years of life.

The term "quality of life" has become a fashionable term to describe a new dimension in health-care delivery, particularly in the arena of catastrophic illness and/or disease. Health-care professionals have readily incorporated into their vocabulary the term "quality of life," as they have incorporated the phrases "treating the whole patient" and "holistic health." A large percentage of the time, health-care professionals use these terms without any notion or ill-conceived notions as to exactly what these terms really mean. But since these terms are part of the currently accepted and expected jargon in the health-care environment, they rattle them off ad nauseam. Health-care professions somehow perceive that if they use these terms they are, in fact, delivering what the terms imply. Nothing could, in fact, be further from the truth.

Quality of Life—A Term or Concept

In reality, the term "quality of life" is a concept, and as such needs to be thoroughly understood if it is to be appropriately put into practical reality.

Twycross[3] has presented a concrete definition of this concept.

> Quality of life refers to the subjective satisfaction expressed or experienced by
> an individual in his/her physical, mental and social situation—Quality of life
> refers to the objective achievement by certain persons of attributes and skills
> that are highly valued in our culture, such as intellectual ability, physical
> capacity, emotional stability, artistic and technical skills, capacity to form and
> enjoy social relationships.

Embodied in this definition are two sub-concepts. They are 1) subjective
satisfaction and 2) objective achievement.

Subjective Satisfaction

Subjective satisfaction refers to the impressions held by a given individual as to
how they view and evaluate their worth and value in life. This sub-concept is
subjective/ideographic and as such is tied closely to the individual's self-esteem,
which is the evaluative component of self-concept.[4] It must be remembered that
any given individual is entitled to their personal view of their worth and value no
matter how inaccurate this view is tied to specific facts or reality.

Should an individual make a statement such as, "I am useless, a burden on my
family and friends and might just as well be dead," this subjective satisfaction
view must be respected and at all accounts must not be disregarded, discounted
or countered. Responses from occupational therapists such as, "I'm sure you
don't really mean that," "You really are a wonderful person, all you need is a
positive attitude," or "You are just making yourself and your family members
more miserable by saying these things," are totally insensitive, irresponsible and
unprofessional.

Objective Achievement

Objective achievements are the real, tangible skills and abilities that a person has
either acquired or learned and can be done with a relative measure of success
and competence-achievement. Objective achievements can be measured against
the facts and principles of reality.

When a person feels good about what they have done in the past and/or
present, it is more than likely that their subjective satisfaction will be one of
useful, hopeful and helpful—a positive sense of self-esteem. When a person does
not feel good about past and/or present achievements, or they are not permitted
to experience positive achievements, it is more than likely that they will feel
helpless, hopeless and/or useless[5], a compromised perception of self-esteem.

Careful attention must be given to the concept of quality of life if one is to
effectively use one's personal and professional self-skills.

Personal Characteristics—Use of Self

Interacting with people with AIDS will require the occupational therapist to
pay particular attention to sensitivity/respect and unconditional regard to their

patients, their family members and/or significant others.

Sensitivity and Respect

By the time the occupational therapist comes into direct contact with the patient, their family members and/or significant others, the patient and frequently the family will have no doubt been exposed to numerous experiences and attitudes (verbal and/or nonverbal) of rejection, alienation, abandonment, disapproval, chastisement for their lifestyle and their subsequent diseased state.

To know that you are going to die long before your normal life expectancy— knowing that you will not have the opportunity to realize your life goals and ambitions is a treat tragedy in itself, but coupled with society's most unacceptable disease, it is the greatest insult and indignity that any person should have to experience.

From the initial personal and professional introductions throughout the entire occupational therapy process, the therapist must make and maintain an absolutely clear statement of non-prejudice about the patient's lifestyle, the consequences that led them to acquiring their disease, and the nature and course of their disease. The occupational therapist must step forward with a sincere and genuine personal and professional attitude of compassion, concern, and objectivity. The following guidelines should be taken under consideration:

1. Be sincere, friendly and welcoming in your introduction.
2. Make casual yet sincere conversation about their home/hospital room to convey that you recognize and respect their possessions and territory.
3. Express verbally and nonverbally your concern for the dilemma that they are facing.
4. Assure the patient, their family members, significant others that you are aware of their medical condition, that you are genuinely sorry that they are suffering, and that you hope you can help them increase their level of independence and/or interdependence toward improving their quality of life.
5. No matter how many or few times you are with them, allow each person an appropriate amount of time and attention to express their needs and concerns.
6. Each time on leaving, make it clear when you will return.

Unconditional Regard

Unconditional regard is an extension of and continuation of sensitivity and respect. The difference is that unconditional regard is an attitude of "no strings attached." The occupational therapist who appropriately conveys unconditional regard makes it clear that the patient does not have to 1) explain or defend their lifestyle or their disease, 2) make any excuses for their previous behavior, 3) apologize for their actions, or 4) make pretenses to make the therapist feel comfortable.

Unconditional regard also implies that the therapist allows the patient, family members, significant others to 1) speak openly and honestly about their present situation and their future; 2) share their concerns, fears, regrets, hopes and wishes without any judgments or advice being given; 3) express their feelings and emotions openly without either them or you feeling embarrassed or uncomfortable.

The unconditional regarding of other people, your patients, as "equal" regardless of their differing beliefs, values and or lifestyles, requires a particular maturity on the part of the occupational therapist. An important principle is a genuine caring and concern for others. Truly caring for and conveying your feelings to them will go a long way to help your patient find some relief, comfort and peace. "Any treatment that does not also minister to the human spirit is grossly deficient."[1]

The Academic Therapist — Bedside Manner

Shaking Hands

The social custom of shaking hands has long been an accepted way of greeting and saying goodbye to people. Shaking hands not only conveys to the patient that you are genuinely pleased to make their acquaintance and that you regard them as a person, but it is also a very effective tool for assessing the patient's self-concept and tolerance for personal (physical) contact.

Use of Names

Every patient-therapist interaction should be professional and businesslike. Although programs can be less formal and structured than traditional health-care agencies, the health professional must never lose sight of the nature of professionalism. It is common protocol to address adult patients by their surname, unless the patient expressly requests being called by his given name. A name is perhaps a person's single most identifying feature and is a key component of self-concept. In acute care facilities it is not uncommon to observe entire patient-therapist interactions in which the patient's name is never used. Such interactions can become sterile and impersonal, and patients may come to believe that the therapist is not truly interested in them, or does not remember who they are or what their needs may be. Appropriate and consistent use of the patient's name conveys two things to the patient:

1. That the therapist remembers the patient's name and shows regard for the individuality of the patient by frequently using his/her name,
2. It helps the patient focus on his part in the patient-therapist interactions. Such personalizing can turn the patient's attention to the interaction and encourage the responsibility to act and react as a person.

The therapist should never assume, no matter what the patient's age, that using first names is in any way appropriate or that using them will facilitate a better relationship between the patient and therapist.

Eye Level Communication

Apart from body stature, eye contact can be the most powerful means of influence. It has been said that they eyes are the window to the soul (personality) of a person. Their position—above or below another—and their physiognomy can clearly make statements of superiority and dominance, concern and compassion, or indifference and superficiality.

Always interact with the patient at eye level. It is not uncommon to expect that the majority of patients will be in bed at the time of admission, and if not in bed, in a chair. If the patient is in bed, never stand over the patient. Because of the nature of the situation, patients are already apprehensive. They may be frightened or panicky as well. Standing over the patient can convey an attitude of superiority, authority and/or dominance which can quickly make the patient feel subservient or vulnerable to "what the professional may be going to do to them."

Guidelines for Eye Contact

1. Following appropriate introductions, pull up a chair and place it three to five feet from the patient's face. If there is no chair, look for a footstool, commode, or wheelchair to sit on.
2. Lower the siderail to eliminate any sense of barriers.
3. Whenever possible, raise the head of the bed so that the patient is in a sitting position, bring the patient to a bedside sitting position, or transfer to or have the patient get into a chair or wheelchair.

Although these may seem like very ordinary procedures, each one can substantially lessen the patient's sense of passivity and intimidation, and can foster an atmosphere of "equal" interpersonal action and communication.

The Physical Examination

When the time comes to examine the patient physically, always tell the patient what you would like to do and why, and ask permission before doing so. An appropriate statement might be, "I would now like to check your arms and legs to see how your muscles and joints are so that you and I can make a plan to increase your independence, is that all right with you?" The therapist is, of course, going to physically examine the patient, but there can be a substantially different relationship between the patient and the therapist in the days to come if the therapist lets the patient know in advance what is to be expected and asks permission. In doing so, a partnership can develop that will strengthen both the patient's self-concept and the therapist's potential.

During the physical examination the therapist must always take special measures to protect the patient's privacy and dignity. Although many patients will say, "It doesn't matter, I got used to losing my dignity in the hospital," there is absolutely no need to "expose" the patient to any indignity or embarrassment while examining and assessing them.

Guidelines for the Physical Examination

1. Before pulling back the bed covers, be certain that the patient is modestly covered, even if it means reaching under the bed covers and arranging pajamas or gowns. (Always remembering to explain to the patient beforehand what you are going to do and to ask permission.) Should the patient refuse a physical examination, listen carefully, ask questions, and assess why the patient is saying no. Although it is important to respect the rights and wishes of all patients, there is also the matter of using time efficiently. The therapist, as well as all other professional team members, must use time to the very best of their ability. Therefore, one cannot afford to comply with every refusal. If the patient is visibly upset, experiencing adverse symptoms, or in obvious distress, the sensitive therapist will ask a few leading questions, assess the general patient and family situation, and make a scheduled appointment to return in a day or two. When patients give a list of excuses that appear to the therapist to be intentional, diversional, or self-fulfilling of misery, the therapist can capitalize on the situation by saying, "I am so sorry that you are feeling so miserable today, let me look you over very quickly so that I can call the doctor. I'm sure there is something that can be done to make you feel more comfortable." Such a statement "feeds into" the patient's immediate needs and allows the therapist to proceed with, at least, a partial assessment.

2. When the patient is ready for the physical assessment and is appropriately covered, the therapist should put down the siderail and ask the patient if it would be all right if you sat on the side of the bed. Doing so puts the therapist in a much better position to perform a manual muscle test and joint range of motion, and allows the therapist to remain at eye level with the patient.

3. During the physical examination the therapist is more than likely to encounter catheter equipment, emaciated extremities, bed sores, or surgical scars. These indignities are far more than a casual concern or embarrassment to the patient—they are the grim reminders of their disease, loss of function and control, and disfigurement. Patients will be fully aware that the therapist is noticing these signs of their illness. Therefore, the sensitive therapist will make casual and caring conversation to ease the situation. No matter how grim the situation may be, the therapist must find and point out the patient's assets and strengths, no matter how minimal they may be. There is no situation where some positive influence, on the part of the occupational therapist, cannot ease the situation and give a glimmer of hope that all is not lost, and that there is a possibility that a measure of independence can be regained.

Eye contact and facial expression during the assessment and physical examination, not only can ease the patient's apprehensions, but also allows the patient to verbalize concerns in a safe and secure environment. Following the physical assessment, the occupational therapist should share his findings with the patient in an honest, straightforward and understandable manner. These findings must be more positive than negative. Following the assessment and physical examination the therapist must give the patient some indication of what goals may be achieved. This gives the patient a clear perception of what will be planned and expected in the days and weeks to come, and, with it, will provide a sense of positive assurance.

Laboratory Exercises For Bedside Manner

One of the most effective ways for the student to learn is first to observe the instructor/therapist in a given situation. Second, hold a discussion in which the student is expected to give a detailed report on the situation and question the instructor on what was done and why. Third, the student "acts" as the therapist with the instructor observing, followed by the instructor giving a detailed report on the student's skills. This procedure is repeated until the student has grasped the essentials of the task being learned. This style of learning will consume a fair amount of time; however, learning "how to" is as important as learning the theoretical information. Students must have both if they are to become reasonably effective entry-level therapists.

It is advised that students not be used to role play patients for two reasons.

1. Students generally do not have the clinical or pathologic knowledge and experience to act out the needs, attitudes and behaviors of a chronically ill adult patient, and therefore, cannot give a sufficiently realistic portrayal to challenge the student/therapist.
2. A student-patient, student-therapist interaction puts each student at a distinct disadvantage because they are friends and peers. The acting of roles, in which both are unfamiliar and uncertain, adds little to appropriate learning.

Therefore, the instructor acts the role of the patient. If one instructor cannot give all students sufficient learning experiences, other faculty members, hospice volunteers or selected community individuals can be used to be "the patient." With the instructor or other unfamiliar adults, the students will experience a measure of stress which more likely will resemble an actual student/patient interaction.

If other instructors or volunteers cannot be organized, the course instructor will have to select four or five class members to act as patients. In this situation, the instructor should develop a wide variety of patient cases and train the students in the behaviors that must be conveyed in the role playing situations. These students then act as patients until the last portion of the course when they will assume the therapist role and the instructor will assume the patient role.

The above procedure will be carried out through subsequent chapters on assessment, treatment planning, and treatment.

Equipment Needed for Exercise
1. Hospital bed
2. Wheelchair
3. Commode
4. Straight back chair
5. Footstool

Environment

A simulated hospital room and a home-like bedroom.

Stage Setting for Exercises

1. Patient wears pajamas or hospital gown in bed with siderails up.
2. Student acts as primary caregiver.
3. Therapist and student knock on door and make introductions.
4. One or two pieces of furniture present in addition to hospital bed.
5. Small group of students observe.

Exercise One

1. Patient is in bed.
2. Therapist introduces self and student to the primary caregiver(s).
3. Therapist introduces self and student to the patient and explains the reason for the visit and the role of the occupational therapist.
4. Patient is relatively compliant.
5. Therapist demonstrates bedside manner techniques while carrying on a casual conversation (10 to 15 minutes); therapist and student make closure with patient and primary care giver(s) and exit.
6. Procedure is repeated with student as therapist; instructor accompanies the student.

Exercise Two

1. Repeat steps 1, 2, and 3 (Exercise One).
2. Patient is non-compliant, withdrawn and avoids eye contact.
3. Repeat steps 5 and 6 (Exercise One).

Exercise Three

1. Repeat steps 1, 2, and 3 (Exercise One).
2. Patient is relatively compliant.
3. Therapist does a gross muscle test and range of motion of upper and lower extremities.
4. Repeat steps 5 and 6 (Exercise One).

References

1. Cousins, N. (1985). *Anatomy of an Illness*. Toronto: Bantam Books, p. 133.
2. Tigges, K.N. and Marcil, W.M. (1988). *Terminal and Life Threatening Illness: An Occupational Behavior Perspective*. Thorofare, NJ: Slack.
3. Twycross, R. (1987). Quality before quantity - A note of caution. *Palliative Medicine*, 1(1):65-72.
4. Miller, J. (1983). Enhancing self-esteem. In *Coping with Chronic Illness*. Philadelphia: F.A. Davis, pp. 275-280.
5. Tigges, K.N. and Marcil, W.M. (1988). *Terminal and Life Threatening Illness: An Occupational Perspective*. Thorofare, NJ: Slack, pp. 124-128.

11 The Occupational Therapy Process

Assessment, Treatment Planning, and Implementation

Kent N. Tigges, MS, OTR, FAOTA, FHIH
William M. Marcil, MS, OTR

If we put together all that we have learned from anthropology and ethnology about primitive men and primitive society, we perceive that the first task of life is to live. Men begin with acts, not with thoughts.

—W.G. Sumner

Introduction

One of our greatest hopes is that we will have good health. We hope and expect that our lives will be safe and secure, comfortable and productive, that we will be happy and considered of value to those we love and care about.

It is far from normal for one to think about or even contemplate being critically ill with the very real fear of dying in the near future. Yes, I am gay. How it happened I do not know—it just did, and became a way of life to me. Believe me, it hasn't been easy to live the life I do, because I know how unacceptable my lifestyle is to you. I have heard you make jokes and tell stories about me and others who live the way we do. You may think it's funny, but believe me, your insensitivity is very hurtful. You may not know it, but I am a professional person. I work hard, do a very good job. I pay my bills and taxes. I go to church, volunteer for several organizations that look after the homeless and abused.

Although I was very familiar with the risks associated with my behavior, I always took special precautions to avoid being infected. Although I know that others have been infected and have died, I never thought it would happen to me.

When I first became ill, I thought it was the flu, a cold, or just one of those bugs that everyone was catching. It never crossed my mind that it was AIDS. You may think me a fool for not thinking I had AIDS, but denial is a very powerful mechanism. When I was told my diagnosis, the initial shock was so devastating that I met it with utter disbelief and denial. "This is really not happening to me. This is a nightmare that will go away!" When it didn't go away, and the grim reality that my life was ruined sank in, I experienced a wide range of reactions. I was angry, resentful, bitter. When I was alone I cried—sobbed my heart out, because I did not want to die. There are so many things that now I will never be able to start or finish. More importantly, I feared of what my family, friends and associates would think of me when they learned I had AIDS. The pain of just thinking about it was unbearable.

Being in the hospital—this is my third admission—is embarrassing and degrading. Why is it that I am always put at the end of the corridor? Why is it that no one ever comes into my room except to give me my medicine? I had always believed that health professionals were a very special breed of people that cared about the sick, injured, disabled and diseased. The days are very long in the hospital. I have no visitors—no telephone calls—only three cards. When a nurse did come into my room, I could feel the cold and distant feelings she held for me. "Take this medicine" was all she ever said to me. I had to bathe myself because the nurses didn't want to touch me. They didn't say that but I knew that was the reason. I once asked if there was an occupational therapist in the hospital that could help me in some way to be more independent. The nurse said she would ask but to not hold my breath. The answer was that the occupational therapy department as well as the physical therapy departments were too busy with their rehabilitation patients. As bad as my physical pain was I could tolerate it. What I could not tolerate was the pain of isolation and abandonment from the very people I thought would give me some care and comfort—the health professionals. I rarely saw my physician in any of my stays in the hospital. I suppose he was also too busy helping people that were going to live.

I guess I am on my own—all by myself to see myself as best I can until I die.
—Anonymous, Philadelphia, January 1990

Occupational Therapy Assessment

Seriously or terminally ill patients, be they advanced cancer or AIDS patients, are not readily welcomed into acute care facilities. This is due largely because hospital personnel are uncomfortable with the diseases and expected outcome—death. In the case of AIDS an added distress is a fear of contracting the disease. As a result these patients are often, if not frequently avoided, and thus neglected, leading the patient to often experience isolation, abandonment and poor health care.

It is extremely important that the occupational therapist be made aware of each and every AIDS patient within the first 24 hours of admission. Physicians or nursing personnel may try to thwart early occupational therapy assessment because they may feel that the patient is too acutely ill and not "ready for rehabilitation." Should this be the case, the occupational therapist must stand firm and present the following arguments:

1. Due to the negative social attitudes toward the disease it is important the patient be made aware that there are other hospital personnel that are concerned about them apart from their direct medical care.
2. Bed rest promotes loss of physical strength and endurance, contractures, poor breathing, urinary tract infections, and bedsores.
3. Being "isolated" promotes personal/emotional feelings of isolation and abandonment—loss of positive self-esteem, depression.
4. Increased activity, no matter how minimal, promotes a stabilizing physical status and is likely to improve the physical status of the patient.
5. Setting goals around increasing independence promotes an attitude of positive well-being and a sense of control and purposefulness.
6. Patients that feel better about themselves are less likely to be demanding of nursing personnel.

As it is likely that acute care physicians and nurses perceive that there is no value or need for rehabilitation services for the AIDS patient. It may be essential for the occupational therapist to explain the nature of palliative rehabilitation.

The term *palliative rehabilitation* is defined as the therapeutic process that promotes temporary restoration and economy of physical potential as it directly relates to the enhancement of potential toward quality of living experiences in occupational roles, that is, increasing muscle strength, endurance, joint range of motion, balance, coordination, ambulation, energy conservation, teaching transfer techniques, wheelchair mobility and use of assistive devices as they relate to preferred personal performance in self-care, work and leisure activities.

The term palliative rehabilitation was first introduced in 1989 by Tigges, in a lecture at the State University of New York at Buffalo, to clarify and differentiate the focus of practice in occupational therapy between acute care, traditional rehabilitation, maintenance and terminal care intervention. Although the skills assessment instruments, goals and treatment process in palliative rehabilitation are the same as those employed in acute care, rehabilitation and the maintenance models, the major exception in palliative rehabilitation is the expected outcome. In terminal care the expected outcome is rapid and progressive physical deterioration resulting in death.

The assessment and treatment process will be effective only if it is founded on a sound model of occupational therapy intervention. With AIDS, as with terminal cancer, the authors have found that the occupational behavior model of practice has been the most effective model of intervention. Figure 11-1 presents selected assumptions and concepts of the occupational behavior model.

Assessment Protocol

On obtaining the necessary physician's referral, the following procedure is to be followed: Review the relevant human growth and development profile of the patient.

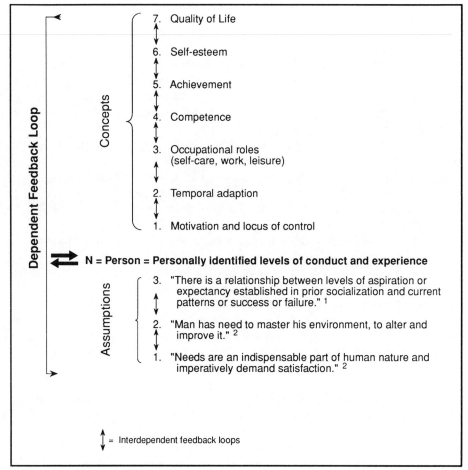

Figure 11-1. Selected Assumptions and Concepts of Occupational Behavior. ©1991, *K.N. Tigges.*

Step 1: The Occupational History

The occupational history (Figure 11-2a-e), is an interview instrument to obtain an overall view of the individual in their past and present roles. The yield of the occupational history is a clear view of the patient as a person—who and what he was, how he previously viewed and valued life, and how he now perceives his present and future goals and expectations. Through the administration of the occupational history a professional, yet personal relationship begins to develop. As the occupational history is informal and inquires about the person's life, the patient rightfully begins to develop trust and respect for the therapist, and as well as a feeling that the occupational therapist is truly interested in him as a person and not just as "another patient." The occupational history goes a long way in developing a strong and sincere relationship that will be so necessary in the patient-therapist interactions. The occupational history assesses the person, temporal adaptation and occupational roles.

Occupational History

Patient's Name _____   Time of History _____

Date of History _____   Age_____

Address _____   Religion _____

Telephone _____   Primary Caregiver _____

Diagnosis _____   Referring Physician _____

Questions   Responses

A. Work History (employment)
1. I understand that before you   _____
   became ill, you were a _____   _____
   What an interesting job! How did   _____
   you get started/interested in that   _____
   line of work?   _____

2. What sort of training/education   _____
   was involved?   _____

3. Where did you get your training?   _____

4. What was the first job you had?   _____
   What jobs did you have after that?   _____

5. What was the last job you had   _____
   before you became ill? What did   _____
   your job actually entail?   _____

6. Did you work up until you got   _____
   sick?   _____

7. (If retired) How long have you   _____
   been retired?
Occupational History, K.N. Tigges, 1986 by the American Occupational Therapy
Association, Inc., Reprinted with permission.

Figure 11-2A.
Occupational
History
Assessment
(employment).
*Figures 11-2a-e
from Tigges,
K.N. and Marcil,
W.M. (1988).
Terminal and
life-threatening
illness: An
occupational
behavior
perspective.
Thorofare, NJ:
SLACK
Incorporated.*

B. Work History (homemaker)

1. I understand that you have   _____
   been a homemaker/parent for   _____
   many years. That is more than   _____
   a full-time job, isn't it?   _____

2. What was the most challeng-   _____
   ing part of being a home-   _____
   maker? A spouse? A parent?   _____

3. What was the most frustrating   _____
   part of being a homemaker? A   _____
   spouse? A parent?   _____

4. Apart from being a full-time   _____
   homemaker, were you ever   _____
   interested or involved in com-   _____
   munity or religious activities?   _____
   If yes, what were they?   _____

5. Were you still active in these   _____
   activities until you became ill?   _____

6. Since you became ill, what   _____
   jobs have been the most dif-   _____
   ficult to give up?   _____

7. What bothers you the most   _____
   about the jobs you have had   _____
   to give up?   _____

8. What type of work is/was   _____
   your spouse involved in?   _____

Figure 11-2B.
Occupational
History
Assessment
(homemaker).

Figure 11-2C.
Occupational
History
Assessment
(family
history).

C. Family History

1. Have you always lived in _____ (city)? If no, where did you live before you moved here?

2. What did your parents do for a living?

3. Do you have brothers and sisters? Where do they live? Do you see/talk to them often?

4. I understand that you have children/grandchildren. Where do they live? Are they married? Do you see talk to them frequently?

5. Before you got sick, what were your duties/responsibilities around the house?

6. Before you got sick, what did you do with your spouse, children, grandchildren, friends, for fun or relaxation?

7. What are the most important things that your illness has prevented you from doing?

8. At the present time what brings you the greatest pleasure?

9. What are the things you would most like to do now?

Work _____

Self-care _____

Leisure _____

Comments _____

Figure 11-2D.
Occupational
History
Assessment
(temporal
adaptation
assessment).

Temporal Adaptation Assessment

Questions

Responses

1. Before you got sick, was it important for you to have a daily schedule? In what way was it important/not important to you?

2. How did you organize your day? Start from the time you got up each morning and tell me everything you did before you went to bed.

3. What is your daily schedule like now?

4. If you had your choice, how would you like to spend tomorrow?

Performance Assessment

KEY: Good = independent
        Fair   = in need of assistance
        Poor = unable to perform

Questions   Strengths------------Deficits
Ask the patient/client to demon-
strate the following:
Bathing   _____
Dressing   _____
Toileting   _____
Mobility   _____
Object manipulation   _____

Home management   _____
Homemaking   _____
Child care   _____
Parenting/grandparenting   _____
Play/leisure   _____

Comments

Figure 11-2E. Occupational History Assessment (performance assessment).

Step 2: Locus of Control-Motivation

The second assessment in the occupational behavior model is locus of control. This assessment reveals the patient's motivational profile. As such the occupational therapist can speculate how the patient will approach both familiar and novel situations and whether the patient feels he is in control of his life or if he feels others control his life (Figure 11-3).

Although there are numerous loci of control assessments, the Reid assessment[4] has been found to be particularly useful (Figure 11-4).

The administration of the locus of control assessment is twofold. The instructions for the first test are: "Please complete this questionnaire as you would have prior to becoming ill." Those for the second text are: "Please complete this questionnaire as you presently feel." A person's perception of their locus of control is highly influenced by their present circumstances and therefore it is essential to obtain a pre-morbid as well as a present perception in order to accurately make a "diagnosis" of actual and perceived motivational profile.

The issue of motivation—locus of control—has long been debated. Many professionals perceive motivation as "what they want or expect the patient to do." If the patient does not do what they want him to do, they report that the patient is "not motivated." Motivation is a much more complex phenomena than "doing or not doing" something. The understanding of why a person will do something in one situation and not another is highly dependent on a variety of factors. Rotter[5] provides a clear definition of the concept of motivation.

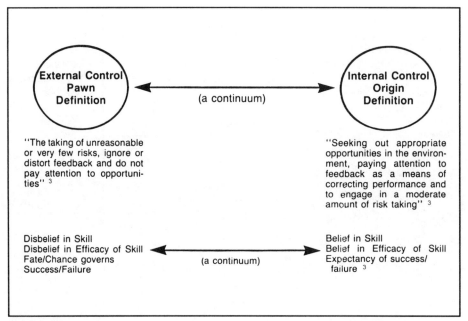

Figure 11-3. Intrinsic Motivation. *Tigges, K.N. and Marcil, W.M. (1988). Terminal and life-threatening illness: An occupational behavior perspective. Thorofare, NJ: SLACK Incorported*

> The potential for a specific behavior to occur in a given situation under circumstances where there are available reinforcements is a function of the expectancy in that situation for an available reinforcement and the value of that reinforcement in that situation.[5]

Step 3: Assessment of Self-Esteem

An effective way to assess self-esteem is to measure it against the loss of self-esteem. The loss of self-esteem is in three descending categories: helpless, hopeless, and useless. Each of these categories has three components. They are 1) observable behaviors, 2) probable causes, and 3) feelings expressed. These categories of loss of self-esteem and their three assessment components are illustrated in Figures 11-5 through 11-7.

The first degree of loss is helplessness. The observable behaviors are
- withdrawal from activity due to fear of additional physical activity
- excessive demands
- diminished ability to control emotions

The probable causes are
- loss of physical strength and endurance
- loss of independence in self-care, work, and leisure
- dependence on medications, catheters, colostomies, etc.

The issue—the problem—is loss of control. When people lose or are denied the opportunity to be in control of their lives, they are likely to react by withdrawing from active engagement in life, and resent or refuse to submit to the

The following are statements which describe either yourself or the beliefs you have.

We emphasize that we are interested in your own opinion, not your judgement of what others think. From time to time you may find that some items seem to be repeated. Don't worry about this, for each item is purposefully different in terms of its specific wording.

Would you please go ahead and rate your degree of agreement or disagreement to each statement by circling the number that best fits your answer for each statement.

	Strongly Agree	Agree	Un-Decided	Disagree	Strongly Disagree
1. People tend to ignore my advice and suggestions.	1	2	3	4	5
2. Maintaining my level of health strongly depends on my own efforts.	1	2	3	4	5
3. It is difficult for me to get to know people.	1	2	3	4	5
4. I can usually arrange to go on outings that I'm interested in.	1	2	3	4	5
5. The situation in which I live prevents me from contacting my family as much as I wish.	1	2	3	4	5
6. I spend my time usually doing what I want.	1	2	3	4	5
7. Although it is sometimes strenuous, I try to do the chores by myself.	1	2	3	4	5
8. I find that if I ask my family (or friends) to visit me, they come.	1	2	3	4	5
9. I have quite a bit of influence on the degree to which I can be involved in activities.	1	2	3	4	5
10. I rarely find people who will listen to me.	1	2	3	4	5
11. My getting away from the house (home) generally depends on someone else making the decisions.	1	2	3	4	5
12. Visits from my family (or friends) seem to be due to their own decisions, and not my influence.	1	2	3	4	5
13. People generally do not allow me to help them.	1	2	3	4	5
14. I can entertain friends when I want.	1	2	3	4	5
15. Keeping in contact with interesting ideas is easy for me to do.	1	2	3	4	5
16. I am able to find privacy when I want it.	1	2	3	4	5

Figure 11-4. Reid locus of control assessment. *Reid, D.W. and Ziegler, M. (1981). The desired control measure and adjustment among the elderly. In H. Lefcourt (Ed.), Research with the Locus of Control Construct, Vol. 1. New York: Academic Press. Used by Permission.*

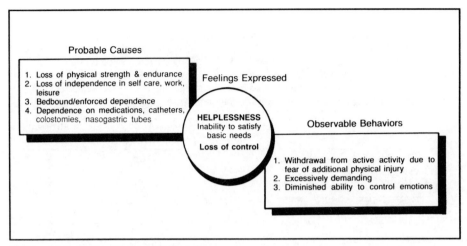

Figure 11-5. Self-esteem: helplessness.

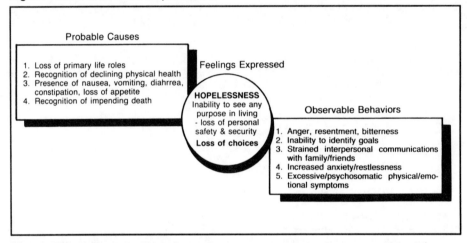

Figure 11-6. Self-esteem: hopelessness.

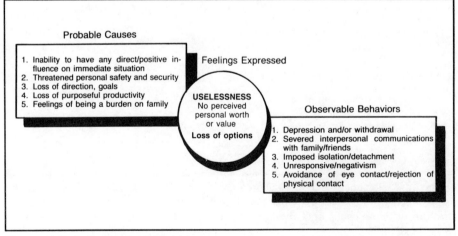

Figure 11-7. Self-esteem: uselessness.

attentions of well-meaning family and staff. Helplessness begins the day that the diagnosis is learned[6] and is compounded by the progressive loss of physical strength and endurance. By nature people are accustomed to being in control of their physical capabilities. One's physical capabilities are the vehicle through which their personal aspirations of competence and achievement are realized. When one's physical abilities become diminished, the emotional and intellectual capabilities become thwarted.

Physical helplessness is perhaps the greatest insult-to-injury that a person can experience, as it occurs abruptly after a state of functional ability. To have one's intellect and mental capabilities intact, yet have to depend on family members and health professionals to hold a glass of water, place a bedpan, prop-up in bed, fluff a pillow, get into a wheelchair, while all the time trying to minimize the gravity of the situation, is a constant and grim reminder that one has lost the capacity to stand on one's own two feet to be free to come and go through life on one's own determination. Helplessness is painful and demeaning. It is the inability to satisfy basic needs. The problem is *loss of control*.

The second degree of loss of quality of life is hopelessness. The observable behaviors and symptoms are
- Anger, resentment and bitterness
- Inability to identify goals
- Strained interpersonal communications with family and friends
- Increased anxiety and restlessness
- Excessive psychosomatic, physical or emotional symptoms
- Noncompliance with medications or therapeutic interventions.
The probable causes are
- Loss of primary life roles
- Recognition of declining physical health
- Presence of nausea, vomiting, diarrhea and constipation
- Recognition of impending death
- Poor or inadequate coping mechanisms prior to illness

The significant problem identified with the state of hopelessness is the *loss of choices*—the inability to see any purpose in living. It is a loss of personal safety and security.

It has been said that one of the greatest indexes of a person's worth and value to society is his work.[7] One's contribution to life is one's past, present and future legacy—it is not only one's livelihood, but also one's stature. "What I do is what I am." An essential concept of living is to be productive and, most importantly, to have that contribution be appreciated and recognized by family, friends and peers. Of all the multiple and complex roles one assumes in life, it is the role of worker/provider that is the most difficult to relinquish.

When one loses or is denied the opportunity to be a vitally productive person, it is not surprising that symptoms (observable behaviors) such as anger, resentment, bitterness, despondency and noncompliance are exhibited. The third and most devastating degree of loss of quality of life is uselessness. The observable behaviors are
- Depression or withdrawal
- Severed interpersonal communications with family and friends

- Imposed isolation, detachment and disengagement
- Unresponsiveness and negativism
- Avoidance of eye contact, rejection of physical contact
  The probable causes are
- Inability to have any direct or positive influence on the immediate or future situation
- Threatened personal safety and security
- Loss of direction, purpose and goals
- Loss of purposeful productivity
- Feelings of being a burden on family members

The problem identified with the state of uselessness is the *loss of options*. When there are no perceived or valued options, and the hope of having any direct or positive influence in life has been lost or taken away by well-meaning family or staff members, the terror and panic of uselessness and burdensomeness are more than justifiable reasons for patients to become severely depressed, withdrawn, and disengaged. In extreme situations, self-imposed exile from life and living have been observed. Hospital staff members need be particularly perceptive to possible thoughts or acts of suicide or homicide.

During the assessment process some patients, because of their difficulty in adjusting to their circumstances, may respond with an unconditional "nothing" to all of the questions, and state that "everything is perfectly all right and there is no need for occupational therapy." This type of response may indicate that the patient is unable, or unwilling, to acknowledge or discuss the situation with the therapist, or that the patient is barricading himself from any outside interference, verbally or nonverbally expressing that he wants to be left alone and not interfered with under any circumstances.

People with AIDS are sometimes so confused and overwhelmed by the magnitude of their situation that they do not know what their feelings really are or how to appropriately express them. They also may feel that the therapist is not capable of listening to their feelings, or may recognize that they themselves cannot cope with their situation.

When the above responses are made, the therapist tries to break the barrier by posing one or more of the following questions to the patient:

- "Are you feeling a sense of helplessness because you have lost so much of your ability to be independent?"
- "You must be feeling very disappointed and, perhaps, angry at having to give up your work because of your illness. It just doesn't seem quite fair, does it?"
- "Losing your ability to be in control of your life must make you feel trapped and hopeless."
- "Having to rely on your family to do even the simplest things must make you feel very dependent. Do you sometimes feel that there is little to live for?"

If the patient responds to these questions with even the slightest positive indication, the therapist can reconstruct the patient's position to one of guarded optimism with the possibility of looking at options. Should the patient continue to state resistance the therapist should acknowledge the patient's position and right to "face life" as he so chooses. The patient should then be assured that if he wishes to change his position, the therapist will always be available.

There is always the possibility that the patient has either misled the therapist, intentionally or unintentionally, or that the therapist has misunderstood the patient. In responding, the patient will say, "No, that is not exactly what I mean/feel." The therapist then re-clarifies through additional questioning, so that an understanding of feelings and attitudes can be reached.

The skilled occupational therapist knows when and how to pose such questions and how to interpret the responses. How patients react and respond depends largely on their pre-morbid intrinsic motivation. Occupational therapists must maintain a keen sense of priority and sensitivity when assessing where patients stand in relationship to their personal crisis.

Step 4: The Physical Assessment

As with the occupational history, before beginning the physical assessment the therapist explains what is to be done and why, and asks the patient's permission. Patients tend to be more cooperative, less fearful and apprehensive, and feel less intruded upon when they know exactly what is expected of them and that their participation is important. A statement such as, "Now that you have told me what your goals are, I would like to check your arms and legs."

There are situations in which the patient or primary caregiver will refuse to comply with the physical assessment, just as he may have done when responding to the questions relating to how the disease or illness has interfered with his life. Reasons may be:

● Not feeling well
● Having pain/discomfort
● Not up to it
● Too sick/weak/tired
● Too much has already happened today

It is possible that one or more of the above reasons are legitimate. The therapist quickly assesses if the patient is having a bad day and makes arrangements to do the assessment another time.

The patient is, perhaps, being non-compliant because he is fearful to "see" how weak and debilitated his body really is, or he is emotionally unprepared to take concrete steps toward increasing functional independence. Similarly, the primary caregiver(s) may be non-compliant with the physical assessment because they obtain secondary gains by having the patient dependent and do not want the therapist to interfere with the situation; are fearful that any level of increased independence of the patient will cause them additional work, effort or attention; are so over-protective that they do not want to "expose" the patient to unnecessary experiences that may lead to false hopes; or are in the process of disengagement from the patient causing them to resist therapeutic intervention because improvement in the patient's functional ability may be equated with an extension of life expectancy. Therefore, during the physical assessment the therapist must explain that occupational therapy intervention will not foster unrealistic goals, or cause the primary caregivers any additional effort or attention. In fact, occupational therapy intervention not only promotes the patient's level of independence and feelings of accomplishment, but also helps to reduce the caregiver's physical responsibilities.

In the majority of cases, a gross physical assessment is performed, the intent being to establish, relatively quickly, the patient's neuromuscular, cognitive and sensory processing strengths and weaknesses. Although the disease process itself may cause significant disabilities in the above areas, the therapist must be aware that secondary weakness and loss of function due to weeks or months of inactivity or immobility are as significant as the pathological concerns.

During the physical assessment the therapist presses the patient to his maximum potential. Gentle, persuasive encouragement from the therapist will generally result in the patient's cooperation. Throughout the assessment, every attempt must be made to draw attention to the patient's strengths and abilities. No matter how grim the situation may be, there are always positive factors that can be capitalized on; this fact is very important for the patient.

Step 5: The Primary Caregiver Assessment

AIDS patients are often abandoned by their immediate family and friends. There are, of course, many family members that do not abandon their son or daughter. In the case of a gay man there is the probability that a lover will remain faithful and continue as the primary caregiver. In these instances there is the possibility of interpersonal conflicts with family members who may also wish to serve as the primary caregiver. The occupational therapist, of course, does not and cannot take a position between family members and the lover. However, the occupational therapist can take a neutral position of support between all parties concerned, and facilitate the very best position for all.

Regardless of who the primary caregiver is, it will be essential that the occupational therapist assess the primary caregiver(s) to ascertain their ability to care for the patient either in the hospital or in the home. Figure 11-8 is the form for the primary caregiver's assessment.

Step 6: Competency, Achievement, and Quality of Life Assessment

Although competency, achievement and quality of life are separate concepts, they are particularly interdependent with each other and therefore must be assessed simultaneously.

Due to the fact that an assessment instrument that directly relates competency, achievement and quality of life in regard to the occupational behavior model of practice did not previously exist, we have integrated the key features of each of these concepts into an organized assessment form. In doing this we believe that the therapist will be in a more sophisticated position to objectively assess, evaluate, and integrate these concepts into the treatment plan. The assessment instrument takes the five components in Jonson's[12] quality of life definition and assesses these components against the key features of competency and achievement (Figure 11-9).

Note that items a, b and c under each quality of life components are objective. The data obtained to address these areas are taken from the occupational history, the locus of control assessment, self-esteem assessment, physical assessment and the primary caregiver's assessment. Item d in each of the categories is the subjective assessment—how the patient actually feels and/or believes

Inquiries	**Comments**
A. 1) How are you managing with the physical care of the patient?	
2) What are the things you are having most difficulty doing for the patient?	
3) What would you like help with in caring for the patient?	
4) How are you coping with your personal life — are you having time to get out and do things that are important for you to do?	
B. Therapist Analysis 1) Is primary care giver pawn-origin orientation?	
2) Does primary care giver have emotional/physical capabilities to a) adapt to a new model of care, b) does primary care giver need support, beyond occupational therapy to cope?	

Figure 11-8. Primary Caregiver's Assessment. *Tigges, K.N. and Marcil, W.M. (1988). Terminal and life-threatening illness: An occupational behavior perspective. Thorofare, NJ: SLACK Incorporated.*

COMPETENCY	ACHIEVEMENT
As measured against competency components: sufficient or adequate behavior to meet demands of occupational roles; attempts to contact and master the environment[8,9]	As measured against achievement components: A specified level of success, attainment or proficiency; ability to solve situations in occupational roles with success/excellence.[10,11]

COMPETENCY

1. **Intellectual ability**
   a. prior to present condition
   b. presently
   c. projected future potential
   d. patient's current perception (subjective satisfaction)
2. **Emotional stability**
   a. prior to present condition
   b. presently
   c. projected future potential
   d. patient's current perception (subjective satisfaction)
3. **Physical capacity**
   a. prior to present condition
   b. presently
   c. projected future potential
   d. patient's current perception (subjective satisfaction)
4. **Artistic, technical, educational professional skills**
   a. prior to present condition
   b. presently
   c. projected future potential
   d. patient's current perception (subjective satisfaction)
5. **Capacity to form, enjoy and maintain social relationships**
   a. prior to present condition
   b. presently
   c. projected future potential
   d. patient's current perception (subjective satisfaction)

ACHIEVEMENT

1. **Intellectual ability**
   a. prior to present condition
   b. presently
   c. projected future potential
   d. patient's current perception (subjective satisfaction)
2. **Emotional stability**
   a. prior to present condition
   b. presently
   c. projected future potential
   d. patient's current perception (subjective satisfaction)
3. **Physical capacity**
   a. prior to present condition
   b. presently
   c. projected future potential
   d. patient's current perception (subjective satisfaction)
4. **Artistic, technical, educational professional skills**
   a. prior to present condition
   b. presently
   c. projected future potential
   d. patient's current perception (subjective satisfaction)
5. **Capacity to form, enjoy and maintain social relationships:**
   a. prior to present condition
   b. presently
   c. projected future potential
   d. patient's current perception (subjective satisfaction)

Key for Competency, Achievement, and Quality of Life Assessment and Evaluation

Prior to present condition: If premorbid rules, skills and roles (Figure 11-10) were appropriate as measured against the person's family, community and subcultural norms and values in regard to competency and achievement, put INTACT. If competency and achievement were not intact, state rules, skills and roles that are affected and give reasons. Refer to American Occupational Therapy Association, Inc. (1989). Uniform Terminology for Occupational Therapy, Second Edition. Rockville, MD:AOTA.

Presently: Intact: (see above description). **Faculty:** Insufficient/inappropriate behaviors to meet the demands of the situation. **At risk:** state roles and reasons. a. Situational: difficulties/problems. Will resolve as conditions improves. Patient requires/does not require therapeutic intervention. b. In jeopardy, requires immediate and acute intervention.

Projected Future Outcome: Based on objective and subjective data state therapeutic potential for: 1. No change/deterioration with intervention. 2. Maintenance with intervention. 3. Improvement with acute/long-term intervention. 4. Restoration of function with acute or long-term intervention.

Patient's current perception: With direct conversation with the patient state the patient's feelings (subjective/objective) about his quality of life prior to present condition, presently and how he sees his future.

Figure 11-9. Quality of life assessment. © 1990, *K.N. Tigges.*

A person's multiple occupational roles are made up of three interdependent systems. These systems are <u>Rules</u>, <u>Skills</u>, and <u>Roles</u>.

$N + 1$ Roles (super system)
$N =$ Skills (system)
$N - 1$ Rules (sub–system)

As these open systems (levels) are interdependent, the laws of hierarchy apply.

1. The complexity of the levels increases upward. The super–system is the most complex and the last to emerge. The sub–system is the least complex and the first to emerge.

2. The higher level depends on the lower, and the lower is directed by the higher.

3. A disturbance or change in the organism at one level affects all levels.

4. The higher level cannot be reduced to the lower. Each level has its own characteristic qualities.

Definitions

<u>N + 1 Roles</u>: The ability to carry out multiple rules and skills appropriately and consistently within a person's social environment.

<u>N = Skills</u>: The individual activities (Bio–medical: personal/emotional social, biological) Bio–social: self care, work, leisure) that make up in part occupational roles. Each skill is made up of a number of sequential steps.

<u>N–1 Rules</u>: A prescribed guide for conduct and action, e.g. instructions.

<u>Conduct (Social)</u>: The rules of social conduct are determined by examining a person's specific social/economic position and norms in regard to self care, work, leisure.

<u>Action (Biological)</u>: The rules (laws) applying to (e.g.) reflex integration, range of motion, gross and fine coordination.

<u>Activity</u>= State of action, quality of being active, physical motion, agility, natural or normal function. An active agent or force.

<u>Occupation</u>: That to which one's time is devoted, or in which one is regularly or habitually engaged. May also suggest what one uses in the company of others. One's regular business or profession.

Figure 11-10. Rules, skills, roles and the skeleton of occupational behavior. ©1990, *K.N. Tigges.*

regarding each of the five components in regard to his life. Data are obtained through direct questioning/conversation with the patient.

Step 7: The Evaluative Process

The evaluative process requires the very best of the occupational therapist's academic and clinical skills. The evaluation of the data obtained from all the assessments requires not only attention to details, but also a sensitive academic attention to the real personal and medical/rehabilitation needs of the patient. Sensitive evaluation also includes those close encounters with the patient in the setting of realistic short-and long-term goals.

In the evaluative process the occupational therapist should take into account the following principles:

1. All patients regardless of their age, illness, disability or any other circumstances, must always be considered as people, first; ill, diseased or disabled, second.
2. All patients must be considered as people whose lives are at risk.
3. All patients have the right to self-determined quality of life.
    a. The patient is always the pivotal initiative in assessment, treatment planning and treatment implementation.
    b. Each patient has the right to specific and detailed ideographic (personal) and nomothetic (disability related) evaluation.
    c. Patient rights must be aligned with their respective responsibilities within their personal, economic and social environment (Figure 11-10).
4. The interdisciplinary treatment plan must be integrated with the other disciplines, as outlined in Figure 9-5.

To illustrate the assessment and evaluative process, the following case study is presented.

Case Study: Jim

Patient Admission Form

Patient's Name ___Jim___   **Age** ___35___   **DOB** 5/03/54

Address _____

_____

Phone Number _____   **Religion** Catholic

Directions to Home _____

Allergies _____Penicillin_____   **Insurance** Medicaid

Primary Caregiver/Family Information Patient lives alone in second floor flat. Patient's family live in area but are not primary caregivers. Patient is cared for by PCA's around the clock.

Primary M.D. _____
Diagnosis ____AIDS, Toxoplasmosis, IDDM, s/p Right CVA, TB____

Life Expectancy ___12 to 18 months___
History ___Toxoplasmosis with cerebral edema resulting in CVA, Recurring herpes, PCP, candidiasis, tuberculosis___

Medications

1) Retrovir 100mg q4h	7) Zovirax 200 mg q8h
2) Principen 500mg q6h	8) Daraprim 25 mg qd
3) Leucovorin Calciu 5 mg BID	9) Metronidazole 500 mg TID
4) Insulin 100 mg q AM	10) Dipenatol q6h
5) Zantac 150 mg BID	11) Nizoral TID (topical)
6) Nystatin 100 mu/ml TID	12) Pentamidine q month

Pain ___Left shoulder on passive movement, frequent headaches___

Anorexia N/A ___Appetite has increased since beginning Retrovir___

Nausea/Vomiting Denies _____

Bowel Dysfunction Frequent diarrhea _____

Skin Integrity Herpes infection of groin/buttocks, pruritis _____

Bladder Dysfunction N/A _____

Edema Left foot and ankle _____

Respiratory Problems   History of PCP, Maintenance pentamidine

Mouth Care   History of oral thrush

Fatigue   Chronic with minimal activity

Emotional   Patient is extremely anxious and angry about his condition. Is afraid of not being in control of his life and of dying a long, painful death.

Family Concerns   Patient lives alone in second story walk-up flat. Patient's family lives in area but are not involved with his care. Patient has around-the-clock home health aides. Patient's mother visits 1-2 times a week to do cleaning, laundry and shopping. Patient's sister-in-law states that she is concerned about his health and well-being and wants the best for him. She would like to see the patient be independent in administering his own insulin q AM instead of the nurse administering it for him. Patient has confided that his sister-in-law is a long-time IVDU.

Occupational History

Patient's Name   Jim   **Time of History**   10:30 AM

Date of History   09/14/89   **Age**   35   **Religion**   Catholic

Address

Telephone   **Primary Caregiver**   HHA Service

Diagnosis   AIDS, Toxoplasmosis, s/p R CVA, IDDM, TB

Work History

Jim had been employed as a certified public accountant in a firm in New Haven, Connecticut for seven years. He stated that he had always enjoyed school and business and math in particular. He was proud of the fact that he was the only one in his family of ten who had received a college degree. He knew that he wanted to be an accountant since he was a sophomore in high school and worked very hard to maintain good grades. He graduated from the State University of New York at Buffalo in 1978 with a BS in Accounting. While in school he worked a variety of jobs, including waiter, cook and shoe salesman. After graduating he moved to New York City where he held his first accounting position in a department store. In 1981, his lover, who worked for an insurance company, was transferred to New Haven. Jim went with him and found a position in a construction firm—a job he maintained until he became ill. His job included overseeing all accounts and preparing tax information. Jim continued to work after being diagnosed with AIDS but was forced to resign following a stroke caused by a toxoplasmosis infection in July 1989. Jim states that the most difficult thing about his current situation is that he is no longer able to work. He feels cheated in that he was the only member of his family to go to college and move away from the inner city and now he has been forced to return to the life he had worked so hard to escape.

Jim did not discuss his personal life in great detail except to say that he had remained with the same lover for five years and is sure that he contracted the disease from him. His lover moved out of their apartment after Jim was diagnosed and has not been heard from since. Because Jim could not receive the emotional support he needed in New Haven, he returned to his hometown to be closer to his family. He currently lives in a second-story flat with no elevator. He has personal care aides (PCA) 24 hours a day.

Jim's parents were sharecroppers who moved to New York shortly before he was born. His mother worked as a domestic and his father was a factory worker. His mother visits regularly and helps Jim with the house work, laundry, shopping and cooking. His father has never been by and Jim rarely talks about him in the present tense. Of his nine siblings, only one sister visits on occasion.

In addition to his job, Jim enjoyed cooking and describes himself as a "gourmet chef." He also was very athletic and enjoyed swimming, basketball and baseball as recreational activities. Now, he says, the only thing that brings him pleasure is watching game shows and soap operas and sports on television. He states that since becoming ill, particularly following his stroke, he is unable to do any of the things that he previously did or enjoyed.

In response to the question, "What are the things you would most like to do now?" he gave the following responses: Work—to return to his job as an accountant. Self-care—to be able to bathe and dress independently every day. Leisure—to be able to cook his own meals, to go swimming, and to play basketball.

Prior to his illness, Jim was a very organized individual and meticulously planned each day in order to maximize his time. During the work week he maintained a rigid schedule and used the weekends for leisure activities. He now spends most of his day in bed, watching television. He states that he would love to take charge of his own life again and not be dependent on others.

Performance Assessment

The results of the performance assessment were as follows: He requires maximal assistance to transfer in and out of bed but can move around in bed independently. Jim is unable to transfer into the bathtub in order to shower. Due to his left-sided hemiplegia and generalized weakness he is unable to wash under his right armpit, his back and his feet. He is unable to dress his lower extremities and requires maximal assist to dress his upper extremities. He requires maximal assist to transfer on and off the toilet but is able to perform all other aspects of toileting independently. He ambulates short distances using a quad cane with contact guard. He wears an ankle-foot orthosis (AFO) to support his left foot during ambulation. For long distances he uses a wheelchair but cannot propel it himself.

Jim is right-handed and is able to manipulate most objects using only one hand. He does have difficulty when attempting to perform tasks that require two hands such as opening medication bottles and buttoning his shirt.

Jim had previously cared for all of his home management needs but is now totally dependent on others to meet his home management needs. He is unable to participate in any of the leisure activities that he previously enjoyed and now watches television all day.

Locus of Control

Results of the Reid assessment[3] revealed that prior to his illness, Jim was a strong origin personality who was in complete charge of his life. Currently, he displays pawn characteristics that were not present pre-morbidly.

Self-Esteem

Based on the therapist's subjective interpretation, Jim is experiencing feelings of helplessness and hopelessness due to loss of control and choices, his inability to satisfy his basic needs, and loss of personal safety and security.

Physical Assessment

Results of the physical assessment are as follows:

Jim is right-hand dominant and has full use of his right side although he exhibits a generalized weakness with (G-) strength and tires easily. The left upper extremity exhibits trace muscle tone proximally with winging of the scapula and a one-finger subluxation at the glenohumeral joint. He complains of a sharp pain in his left shoulder when it is moved. Distally, he exhibits increased flexor tone with a flexion synergy noted. He has no functional use of his left arm.

Jim is able to bear 50 percent weight on his left lower extremity during transfers and ambulation. He has no active dorsiflexion of his left ankle and must use an AFO to support his left foot during ambulation.

Jim's trunk balance in sitting is good although he requires assistance to come to a sitting position. He has fair standing balance and uses a quad cane when standing and ambulating.

Jim displays no cognitive impairments, is alert and oriented to person, place and time and has no memory or comprehension difficulties. A sensory examination reveals no sensory deficits.

Jim currently has an active herpes infection in his groin and buttocks which makes sitting difficult and painful. He also has a fungal infection of his hands and arms which itches but does not impair his function. He is currently on medications to resolve these conditions.

Primary Caregiver Assessment

Because Jim lives alone and his family is not present on a daily basis, the primary caregiver assessment was directed at the both the day and evening home health aides. Both aides state that they feel somewhat uncomfortable working with Jim because of his disease and state that they know very little about AIDS except what they learned from their one day orientation training. The therapist noted that although they try not to touch Jim unless absolutely necessary, they do not wash their hands before contact or wear gloves when changing dressings on his buttocks.

Both aides state that all transfers are difficult and moving Jim up and down the stairs is extremely difficult.

Exercise for Case Study

Based on the above information, the student will evaluate the data presented and determine what should be addressed in the areas of physical functioning, work, self-care and play/leisure. Consider how the patient can gain competence, achievement, self-esteem, and quality of life in each of these areas.

For each item in the evaluative process, develop short- and long- term goals (with a time frame for each) and state how these goals contribute to an enhancement of competence, achievement, self-esteem and quality of life.

Indicate your proposed treatment schedule (frequency, duration and session length), what the role of the OTR and the COTA will be, describe what will be done to achieve each goal, and what equipment will be necessary. The results of the quality of life evaluation for this case study are presented in Figure 11-11.

The Evaluative Process

Physical Functioning

Strengths: Jim is right-handed and his right-side function is intact, except for loss of strength and endurance. He displays no sensory deficits or cognitive impairments. Static and dynamic trunk balance are good and he is able to bear weight on his left lower extremity.

*Weaknesses:*No functional use of the left upper extremity due to increased tone and flexor synergy. Subluxation of left shoulder with pain on passive movement. Low physical endurance to activity. Unable to sit in wheelchair for long periods of time due to pressure on herpes lesions.

Self-care

Strengths: Able to assist in upper extremity bathing and dressing activities. Independent in toileting activities, except for transfers. Independent in bed mobility.

Weaknesses: Dependent in all transfers. Dependent in lower extremity dressing and bathing. Unable to prepare meals due to low endurance, left hemiparesis and decreased right-sided strength. Difficulty with fastenings and manipulation of medication containers.

Work

Strengths: All cognitive functioning intact. Desired work activities can be performed using one-handed techniques, ergonomics and energy conservation techniques. Speaks articulately in person and on telephone.

Weaknesses: Decreased endurance and short life expectancy, combined with lack of employment contacts in the area make it unlikely that Jim will find regular employment. Unable to perform any home management activities due to limited strength, endurance and mobility. Unable to prepare meals.

Play/Leisure

Strengths: Has interest in activities such as swimming, basketball and baseball.

Weaknesses: Unable to participate in activities due to weakness, low endurance

COMPETENCY	ACHIEVEMENT
As measured against competency components: Sufficient or adequate behavior to meet demands of occupational roles; Attempts to contact and master the environment.[8,9]	As measured against achievement components: A specified level of success, attainment or proficiency; ability to solve situations in occupational roles with success/excellence.[10,11]

1. **Intellectual ability**
   a. **prior to present condition** Intact. Above-average intelligence to meet demands of occupational roles.
   b. **presently** Intact. Above-average intelligence to meet demands of occupational roles.
   c. **projected future potential** At risk. Possible deterioration which could interfere with role behavior.
   d. **patient's current perception (subjective satisfaction)** Patient states that he feels competent but will not be able or allowed to exercise his competency. Feels helpless.
2. **Emotional stability**
   a. **prior to present condition** Intact.
   b. **presently** At risk: symptoms of depression and isolation are present.
   c. **projected future potential** Unknown at present. Predict homeostasis.
   d. **patient's current perception (subjective satisfaction)** Patient expresses helplessness due to inability to meet basic needs.
3. **Physical capacity**
   a. **prior to present condition** Intact.
   b. **presently** at risk (see physical assessment: Cannot exercise competence in former occupational roles.
   c. **projected future potential** Restoration and economy of physical potential with acute intervention.
   d. **patient's current perception (subjective satisfaction)** Patients states he does not feel that any improvement in his physical condition will lead to competence to meet occupational roles.

1. **Intellectual ability**
   a. **prior to present condition** Intact. Above-average intelligence to meet demands of occupational roles.
   b. **presently** Intact. Above-average intelligence to meet demands of occupational roles.
   c. **projected future potential** At risk. Possible deterioration which could interfere with role behavior.
   d. **patient's current perception (subjective satisfaction)** Patient states that he feels competent but will not be able or allowed to exercise his competency. Feels helpless.
2. **Emotional stability**
   a. **prior to present condition** Intact.
   b. **presently** At risk: symptoms of depression and isolation are present.
   c. **projected future potential** Unknown at present. Predict homeostasis.
   d. **patient's current perception (subjective satisfaction)** Patient expresses helplessness due to inability to meet basic needs.
3. **Physical capacity**
   a. **prior to present condition** Intact.
   b. **presently** at risk (see physical assessment: Cannot exercise competence in former occupational roles.
   c. **projected future potential** Restoration and economy of physical potential with acute intervention.
   d. **patient's current perception (subjective satisfaction)** Patients states he does not feel that any improvement in his physical condition will lead to competence to meet occupational roles.

Figure 11-11. Quality of life assessment: Case study.

COMPETENCY	ACHIEVEMENT

4. Artistic, technical, educational and professional skills
  a. **prior to present condition** Intact.
  b. **presently** at risk due to unemployability.
  c. **projected future potential** Improvement with acute intervention.
  d. **patient's current perception (subjective satisfaction)** Intact. Above-average intelligence to meet demands of occupational roles.
5. Capacity to form, enjoy, and maintain social relationships
  a. **prior to present condition** Intact (except for some family stress due to the lifestyle)
  b. **presently** at risk due to lack of social interaction (isolation/abandonment).
  c. **projected future potential** Improvement with acute intervention/socialization.
  d. **patient's current perception (subjective satisfaction)** Patient states that he feels abandoned by everyone.
	4. Artistic, technical, educational and professional skills
	  a. **prior to present condition** Intact.
	  b. **presently** at risk due to unemployability.
	  c. **projected future potential** Improvement with acute intervention.
	  d. **patient's current perception (subjective satisfaction)** Intact. Above-average intelligence to meet demands of occupational roles.
	5. Capacity to form, enjoy, and maintain social relationships
	  a. **prior to present condition** Intact (except for some family stress due to the lifestyle)
	  b. **presently** at risk due to lack of social interaction (isolation/abandonment).
	  c. **projected future potential** Improvement with acute intervention/socialization.
	  d. **patient's current perception (subjective satisfaction)** Patient states that he feels abandoned by everyone.

Figure 11-11. Continued.

and hemiparesis. Unable to access resources in the community.

Treatment Process

After reviewing assessment data, determining strengths and weaknesses and discussing the treatment plan with Jim and his home health aides, the following treatment plan was implemented:

Physical Functioning

1. Short-term goals (1-2 weeks)
   a. Increase right upper extremity (RUE) strength to (G) overall using one pound wrist weights with progressive increase in repetitions. Strength will also be increased by participation in transfers, other self-care activities, and leisure activities
   b. Reduce left upper extremity (LUE) subluxation via subluxation sling and proprioceptive neuromuscular facilitation (PNF) techniques
   c. Fabricate left resting hand splint
   d. Increase patient's sitting comfort in wheelchair by providing gel cushion
   e. Increase patient's comfort in bed by providing water mattress
2. Long-term goals (3-5 weeks)

a. Increase RUE strength to (G/N) overall
b. Normalize LUE muscle tone
c. Increase endurance to moderate activities to 15 minutes
3. Goals for home health aides
   a. Instruct in proper positioning of LUE to normalize tone and reduce subluxation and shoulder pain
   b. Educate aides about modes of HIV transmission and universal precautions
   c. Instruct in proper transfer techniques
4. Goal Objectives: By allowing Jim to increase his physical strength and endurance in a safe and controlled environment, he will be given more control and options, thus increasing his self-esteem by reducing his feelings of helplessness and hopelessness. By allowing him to contact and master his environment, competency can be facilitated, leading to feelings of achievement.

Self-care
1. Short-term goals (1-2 weeks)
   a. Jim will be independent in toilet transfers using assistive devices
   b. Jim will transfer into and out of the bathtub with minimal assist and use of assistive devices
   c. Jim will independently dress his upper extremities each A.M.
2. Long-term Goals (3-5 weeks)
   a. Jim will perform tub transfers with supervision only
   b. Jim will transfer from bed to wheelchair with contact guard only
   c. Jim will transfer into and out of a car with minimal to moderate assist (interdependent)
   d. Jim will perform wheelchair to pool transfers with moderate assist (interdependent)
   e. Jim will don sweatpants with occasional minimal assist at least three days per week.
3. Goal objectives: Perhaps the greatest indignity of any disease or disability is that of being forced into a role of dependence on others to perform the basics of one's own self-care. The inability to meet one's basic needs leads to a sense of loss of control—the hallmark of helplessness. When one is able to have some degree of control in self-care skills, it is likely that one will develop sufficient behaviors to meet the demands of other situations (competence), including work and play/leisure activities.

Work
1. Short-term goals (1-2 weeks)
   a. Jim will contact local accounting agencies by telephone to inquire about part-time or per diem employment
   b. Depending on his physical condition, Jim will assist in the preparation of all meals by choosing the menu, writing a grocery list, and performing rudimentary preparation such as washing and peeling vegetables
   c. Jim will sort his laundry prior to the aides taking it to the laundromat

2. Long-term goals (3-5 weeks)
    a. Jim will formulate a household budget according to his monthly medicaid income
    b. Jim will prepare a simple lunch by himself at least two times per week
    c. Jim will assist in meal clean-up and dish washing tasks at least three times per week
3. Goal objectives: Work is the greatest single index of a persons worth and value to society.[7] Persons with chronic diseases or disabilities are generally not viewed as valuable to society. Persons with AIDS, it would appear, are perceived to be even less valuable, in terms of contribution to society. Work is the focus of Jim's life. By enabling him to participate in some of the work activities that are important to him, his self-esteem will be further bolstered by providing him with even more control and choices in his life and allowing him

Play/Leisure

1. Short-term goals (1-2 weeks)
    a. Jim will identify and participate in one leisure activity per day for thirty minutes, which does not include television
2. Long-term goals (4-6 weeks)
    a. Jim will swim once a week at the local YMCA
3. Goal objectives: Healthy individuals maintain a balance of self-care, work, and play/leisure activities. Both play and work can facilitate and strengthen achievement behavior[2] and therefore they must be employed in balance if effective treatment outcomes are to occur. Swimming, Jim's choice in leisure activities, will allow him to contact and master his immediate environment and gain feelings of success. This activity can allow further increases in physical strength and endurance and thus, promote additional control and choices in other areas of his life.

Treatment Implementation

Due to the number of goals agreed on, it was felt by both Jim and the therapist that the short-term goals would be staggered over seven days of the week. The goals were written down on a calendar to help Jim to remember what needed to be done and to allow him to set daily goals for himself. It was felt that the bio-social goals of work, self-care and play/leisure could be better achieved if the biomedical problems were addressed first.

During the first week, Jim was provided with a subluxation sling to support his left arm which also reduced the subluxation and pain. A resting hand splint was fabricated to maintain a functional position of his wrist and hand. He was also supplied with a gel cushion for his wheelchair to reduce pressure on his buttocks and a wheelchair armrest to properly position his left arm while he was in the wheelchair. The therapist explained to Jim that although he would work with his left arm to regain function, there were no guarantees that he would get any function back. Jim acknowledged this but said that he would hope for the best. He was also given progressive resistive exercises (PRE) for his RUE, as well as instruction in one-handed techniques and dexterity exercises.

By the second week, Jim was feeling confident enough to begin some of his other short-term goals. He began calling about possible jobs in his field but had no luck. Although somewhat disheartened by his lack of success, he made inquiries on a daily basis. After three weeks, the therapist suggested that Jim call the local AIDS council to inquire about employment. Although they could not afford to hire him, they offered Jim a volunteer position doing some book work for the council as well as for other clients. Jim agreed to this arrangement.

After Jim and his aides were comfortable with transfers, he was out of bed every day and began to take a more active role in his daily living skills, including his laundry and meal preparation activities. As he became more adept at using only his right hand in activities, he discovered that he was able to perform some of his former roles, he became more confident and was eager to attempt additional aspects of his home management.

Jim continued to require minimal assistance to transfer in and out of the tub but accepted assistance to shower on a daily basis. With the aid of grab bars, he became independent in toilet transfers. An overhead swivel trapeze was obtained to increase Jim's transfers in and out of bed. He was instructed in one-handed techniques for lower extremity dressing using a dressing stick and a sock-aide.

Due to the increase in activity and because Jim's endurance fluctuated from day to day, he opted to read in bed each afternoon and evening. He also began to keep a journal of his illness and the progress that he was making in gaining back his independence.

The therapist made arrangements with the YMCA to take Jim swimming every two weeks. Because these sessions would take a great deal of time, it was agreed that the therapist would attend the first two sessions and assist both Jim and his aide. In order to get Jim to the pool, it was necessary to instruct Jim and the aide in stair negotiation (together with the physical therapist), car transfers and pool transfers.

At the end of nine weeks, Jim was able to transfer into and out of bed independently with the assistance of the trapeze. He required assistance for tub transfers and became independent in toilet transfers. He was able to shower with minimal assist at least five or six mornings per week. He was able to dress himself completely with the exception of donning his AFO and left shoe. He also required occasional assist with small buttons.

Jim planned all meals and made the grocery list each week. He prepared his own lunch five times per week and cooked an occasional Sunday dinner for family and friends. He assisted in meal cleanup by clearing the table and transporting items on a wheeled cart.

Although the flexor tone in his LUE was inhibited through positioning and other techniques, Jim did not progress beyond this stage and had no functional use of his left arm. However, the subluxation was successfully reduced and the shoulder pain was eliminated. Jim's RUE became stronger (G/N) and he was better able to utilize it during activities.

Through the AIDS council, Jim was able to perform two to three hours of accounting work per week. This work was delivered to his apartment and picked up when it was completed.

Jim's favorite activity was his weekly swimming session which he looked forward to with great anticipation. It was found to be too difficult for the aide to handle alone and Jim was provided with a "buddy" from the AIDS council to help out. A certified occupational therapy assistant also accompanied Jim on these weekly outings. Jim found that he could move easier in the pool and enjoyed his freedom from gravity. Because Jim was anemic, he became cold easily, even in the heated pool, and could not stay in for long periods of time. A short neoprene wetsuit was obtained to help keep him warm while in the pool.

While at the YMCA, Jim renewed his interest in basketball and would spend time shooting baskets from his wheelchair after swimming.

Treatment Results

After nine weeks of therapy, Jim had achieved all of his goals with the exception of normalization of tone in his left arm. Although he did not regain any function in his left arm and he continued to be interdependent and dependent in many areas of self-care, Jim was pleased with the progress that he had made in such a short time. After reviewing the goals, energy conservation and safety techniques with Jim, his aide and his buddy, Jim was discharged from therapy.

Assessment of Quality of Life: A Subjective/Objective Review

Although Jim was initially skeptical and pessimistic about his capabilities, it soon became evident to him that he still had the ability to take control of his life. Each small success and gain gave him increased feelings of competency and achievement which, in turn, gave him further impetus to attempt new tasks. He began to take a more active role in his daily activities even if he could not physically perform some of them.

Despite the progress that he made, Jim still had "bad days" when he was unable to get out of bed or do much for himself. He took these days in stride and would plan his next days activities when he would be feeling better. Jim never lost sight of his disease and realized he would never be the same as he used to be. However, he looked forward to the challenges of each new day with great anticipation. In this case, quality of life was restored.

References

1. Reilly, M. (1962). Occupational therapy can be of one of the greatest ideas of 20th century medicine. *American Journal of Occupational Therapy*, 16(1):1-9.

2. Reilly, M. (1969). The education process. *American Journal of Occupational Therapy*, 23(4):299-307.

3. Kielfohner, G. and Burke, J. (1985). Components and determinants of human occupation. In G. Kielhofner (Ed.) *A model of human occupation*. Baltimore: Williams and Wilkins.

4. Reid, D. The desired control measure: Some psychometric data. Unpublished manuscript. Department of Psychology, York University, Downsview, Ontario, Canada.

5. Rotter, J.B. (1954). Generalized expectancies for internal versus external control of reinforcement. *Social Learning and Clinical Psychology*, 80(1):1-28.

6. Sourkes, B. (1987). Views of the deepening shade. *American Journal of Hospice*

Care, 4(3):22-29.

7. Gregory, I. and Smeltzer, D. (1983). *Psychiatry*. Boston: Little, Brown, pp. 144-145.

8. White, R. (1971). The urge towards competency. *American Journal of Occupational Therapy*, 25(6):271-274.

9. Wolman, B.B. (1973). *Dictionary of Behavioral Sciences*. New York: Van Nostrand Reinhold.

10. Chaplin, J.P. (1975). *Dictionary of Psychology* (rev. ed.). New York: Dell.

11. English, H.B. and English, A.C. (1958). *A Comprehensive Dictionary of Psychological and Psychoanalytical Terms*. New York: McKay.

12. Jonson, A.L., Seigler, M. and Winslade, W.J. (1982). *Clinical Ethics: A Practical Approach to Ethical Decisions in Clinical Medicine*. London: Bailliere Tindall.

Suggested Readings

Bateson, G. (1985). A theory of play and fantasy. *Psychiatric Research Notes*, 2:39-51.

Charlesworth, J. (Ed.) (1964). Leisure in America: Blessing or curse. *The American Academy of Political and Social Science,* 7(96):4.

Marcil, W. and Tigges, K. (1986). The role of the OTR and COTA in hospice care. In S. Ryan (Ed.). *The Certified Occupational Therapy Assistant: Roles and Responsibilities*. Thorofare, NJ: SLACK, pp. 255-267.

Tigges, K.N. (1983). Occupational therapy in hospice. In C.A. Corr and D.M. Corr (Eds.). *Hospice Care: Principles and Practice*. New York: Springer, pp. 164-167.

Tigges, K.N. (1986). Occupational therapy in hospice care. In L. Davis (Ed.). *Role of Occupational Therapy with the Elderly*. Rockville, MD: American Occupational Therapy Association, pp. 261-264.

Tigges, K. and Marcil, W. (1986). Maximizing quality of life for the housebound patient. *American Journal of Hospice Care*, 3(1):21-23.

Tigges, K.N. and Sherman, L.M. (1983). The treatment of the hospice patient: From occupational history to occupational role. *American Journal of Occupational Therapy*, 37(4):235- 238.

Tigges, K.N., Sherman, L.M. and Sherman, F.S. (1984). Perspectives on pain of the hospice patient: The roles of the occupational therapist and physician. *Occupational Therapy in Health Care*, 1(3):55-56.

Trombly, C.A. (Ed.) (1984). *Occupational Therapy for Physical Dysfunction*. Baltimore: Williams & Wilkins.

12 AIDS Facts and Implications for Occupational Therapy

William M. Marcil, MS, OTR

Whatever you cannot understand, you cannot possess.

—Goethe

Introduction

As diseases go, AIDS is a neophyte in the history of medicine and epidemiology. Although much has been learned about AIDS in ten years, there is still much more to be known. What is disturbing about the present situation is that despite our current knowledge about the disease, there are still many within the health-care community that remain ignorant about AIDS and HIV. The authors have noted that in AIDS lectures and in-service training sessions since 1985, many of the same questions continue to be asked about the disease—questions that should not need to be asked based on the extensive wealth of information that is available to the general public. With this in mind, we present here some basic facts about AIDS that should be known by all. Although some may criticize the following information as "AIDS 101," we feel that it is important for one to understand the basics before one can gain further knowledge. Certainly, it is impossible to understand trigonometry if one has no knowledge of algebra. The same argument can be used here as well. Throughout the chapter are implications that we feel are specific to occupational therapists in working with a patient with AIDS/HIV. The field of AIDS is very young and there is much room for alterations and improvements.

Human Immunodeficiency Virus

When individuals began to exhibit the symptoms that we now know as AIDS, the cause of this disease process was unknown. It was not until 1984—three years after the first official cases were noted—that the culprit was unmasked. AIDS is caused by a virus—specifically a retrovirus. All viruses lack the means to reproduce and therefore, by and of themselves, cannot be considered true living organisms. To achieve replication viruses rely on living host cells to provide what they themselves lack. Many viruses contain DNA and utilize the host cell's DNA as a template for DNA replication. The immune system produces antibodies to rid the body of the invading organisms and therefore most viral infections are self-limiting. Antibiotics are not effective in treating viral infections and are not administered unless there is an accompanying bacterial infection.

HIV is unique in a number of ways and, due to these idiosyncrasies, has defied scientists in their search for a cure and/or vaccine. HIV belongs to a class of viruses known as *retroviruses*, which also includes those associated with certain types of leukemia. Retroviruses contain RNA only, but are able to transcribe this RNA into a DNA template of the host cell in a reaction catalyzed by an enzyme called reverse transcriptase, which the viruses bring with them into the cell.[1]

HIV appears to have an affinity for cells that contain a molecule called CD4 as part of their cellular membrane. These cells include T4 helper lymphocytes which are the first line of defense in an immune response, and neuroglia of the CNS, which serve as support cells for neurons, among others.

The T4 helper cells are typically the initial target of HIV. Under normal circumstances the T4 cells seek out invading organisms and alert the immune system to respond. It is ironic that HIV is attracted to the cell it should fear the most.[2] Once the virus has attached to and injected itself into the host, it can remain dormant for an extended period of time before becoming active. Antibodies for HIV are produced in minute quantities initially and may take anywhere from three weeks to three months before they are fully established. This presents a dilemma for those wishing to be tested for the virus. For example, an individual who has been sexually assaulted on Friday night may be tested for HIV infection on Monday morning. Providing that the individual was HIV-negative before the attack, the test will probably be negative. This is because the current tests for HIV only test for the antibodies to the virus—not for the virus itself—and the antibodies may not yet be formed or in great enough numbers to be detected. Therefore, worried individuals should wait three to eight weeks before the initial test, with a follow-up test in three to six months.

How and why the virus becomes activated is not clearly understood at this time. Theories are many concerning activation and range from the presence of certain other "trigger" viruses such as hepatitis B virus (HBV), to poor overall health, to stress. Once activated, however, HIV begins its process of RNA-DNA transcription to replicate. As more new viruses are produced, utilizing the host's organelles, the host eventually becomes exhausted and dies, bursting and releasing the multitude of new viruses to search for new host cells in which to continue the cycle. This causes a domino effect within the immune system and decreases its effectiveness in preventing infection. When the immune response is impaired or absent, the body is made vulnerable to a host of opportunistic infections which will flourish in an unchecked environment. It is the opportunistic infections, many of which are ubiquitous but benign in the presence of a properly functioning immune system, which plague and kill its victims; HIV merely unlocks the gate. For a description of the most common opportunistic infections associated with AIDS, refer to Appendix D.

Persons at Risk for HIV Infection

Viruses cannot think or reason; they merely act on the immediate environment in search of a host cell. If none are available, the virus cannot replicate and will remain benign and eventually die. In this manner, HIV is no different. It must have a host in which to proliferate. The host cells that HIV requires are seemingly unique to humans and therefore we are all at potential risk for contracting HIV infection and subsequently AIDS. However, HIV is difficult to contract and transmission can only occur through intimate contact with an infected individual. Certain groups have been designated as being at extremely high risk for HIV infection. It should be noted that these individuals have been infected by the most intimate of human contact in the absence of precautions. HIV can only be spread through the exchange of blood, semen, vaginal secretions and breast milk.[3] Each of these fluids contain an abundance of lymphocytes—the primary host cell for HIV.

Sexually Active Individuals

Homosexual men are considered by many to be at the highest risk for HIV infection. Statistically gay men comprise 60 percent of all current U.S. cases of AIDS.[4] This does not imply that all gays have AIDS. The reason for the high incidence in this group is primarily due to multiple partners in unprotected sexual relationships. Anal intercourse with an infected individual is an extremely high-risk practice especially if no condom and spermicide is used. The anus was not designed by nature to receive foreign objects. Any trauma can result in rectal tears and bleeding allowing a conduit for HIV infection by way of semen and/ or blood. Preexisting conditions such as hemorrhoids and gonorrhea may also facilitate transmission in this manner. An increased awareness among gay men about safe sex practices and an increased willingness to participate in safe sex has resulted in a decrease in new cases of HIV infection as well as other venereal diseases in this population. However, the use of a condom does not remove all risk of HIV infection and it is best to know one's partner's HIV status.

Although heterosexuals comprise only 5 percent of AIDS cases, it is probable that the numbers will grow in the near future if multiple unprotected sexual encounters occur. Vaginal intercourse is safer than anal intercourse, as the vagina was designed to accommodate the penis and serve as the birth canal. However, fissures and tears, however minute, do occur in vaginal intercourse and can allow entry of HIV. For this reason, it is possible that a woman could contract HIV from an infected man easier than an uninfected man could contract it from an infected woman. Unless one is in a monogamous sexual relationship with an uninfected partner, a condom should be used in conjunction with nonoxydil-9, a spermicide that has been demonstrated to kill HIV. A diaphragm by itself will not protect a woman from HIV infection but it may help to protect the neck of the cervix from trauma and serve as a barrier to HIV. A combination of all three will reduce the possibility of not only HIV infection, but also other venereal diseases and unwanted pregnancies, as well.

While condoms greatly reduce the possibility of contracting HIV and other venereal diseases, they are not the be-all and end-all of protection. There are certain precautions that one must exercise in using a condom to increase its effectiveness. Only latex condoms should be used as the membranous type can allow passage of the virus.[5] The condom should be applied before insertion of the penis in or around an orifice and removed and disposed of immediately following ejaculation. It is recommended that two condoms be used during anal intercourse due to the increased possibility of breakage. Only water-based lubricants such as K-Y jelly should be used with a condom. Other lubricants such as vaseline, which has a petroleum base, can compromise the integrity of the condom.[5] Extremes of temperature and pressure can cause the condom to break down and therefore they should not be stored in wallets, purses or automobiles for extended lengths of time.[5]

Oral intercourse, be it heterosexual or homosexual, appears to be less risky than anal or vaginal intercourse but should be performed with caution. Although the mouth is durable and supplied with a high concentration of immunologic defense mechanisms, it is possible that HIV infection can occur in this manner. Tiny cuts in and around the mouth (from gum disease, brushing or flossing, canker sores or cold sores) can allow HIV to gain access to their hosts. Therefore, fellatio should be performed with a condom and cunnilingus should be performed using a dental dam to reduce the possibility of infection. Anilingus is not considered to be a safe activity and should not be practiced with one of unknown HIV status.

Although HIV has been demonstrated in the saliva of infected individuals, it is not a mode of transmission.[3] As there are no lymphocytes in saliva the virus has no host and is inactivated by the presence of antibodies as well as an acidic environment which is hostile to the virus. Therefore, dry kissing is a safe activity and wet kissing, which is considered to be slightly risky, is also relatively safe. Some persons may engage in other sexual practices in lieu of actual intercourse. These practices may appear safe when in fact they are not. Activities such as fantasy, touching and massage are extremely safe indeed. Mutual masturbation is safe provided that there is no unbroken skin to allow entry of HIV. Masturbation or urination on unbroken skin is also a safe activity. Masturbation onto broken skin (cuts, scrapes, eczema, severe acne, etc.) is not safe and should be avoided. "Fisting," the act of inserting one's hand into another's rectum, is also considered to be a high-risk activity and should not be engaged in. Regardless of the type of sexual activity in which one engages, the participants should wash their hands and genitals before and after sexual contact.

For all sexually active persons outside of a monogamous relationship and when the partners HIV status is not known, safe sex guidelines should be strictly followed. The best deterrent to HIV is abstinence. When this is not an option, one should assume that any potential sexual partner is HIV-positive and act accordingly.

Intravenous Drug Users

IVDUs comprise 21 percent of the current U.S. AIDS cases.[4] This group is at risk primarily by direct contact with infected blood by way of sharing needles. Many drug users may be aware of the dangers associated with sharing needles but their fear of contracting AIDS or other diseases such as hepatitis is overridden by their addiction and their need to get their next "fix." Interviews with recovering addicts[6] reveal the obsession with the drug and the overwhelming desire to get high. Within a "shooting gallery," the user injects the drug into a vein and then draws back on the plunger until blood enters the needle. The mixture of drug and blood is then re-injected. This process is often repeated many times before the user passes the needle on to the next individual. Each person who performs this ritual passes minute quantities of their blood to all participants. If, in a shooting gallery of seven individuals, the first person to use the needle is HIV-positive, the other six will inevitably contract the virus through that needle.

It should be noted that it is not the drug that passes the virus, it is the vehicle in which it is transported. One can snort cocaine and never have to worry about contracting HIV (although the cocaine may impair the individual's judgment leading to other high-risk behaviors). However, if the cocaine is injected and the needle is shared, then there is the possibility of infection. Similarly, today there is an obsession with body building and anabolic steroids are often used as a shortcut to a perfect body. By injecting the steroids and sharing the needles, the part-time body builder is at much risk for HIV infection as the full-time junkie.

To prevent HIV infection in this manner, IV drug users must be educated to not share their needles and/or clean the needles before and after each use in a bleach solution, which will kill the virus.

Recipients of Infected Blood and Blood Products

Prior to 1985 there was no way to tell if blood used in transfusions was infected with HIV and many individuals became infected by the same blood that had saved their lives. While engaging in unprotected sex or sharing needles puts one at extremely high risk of contracting HIV, the receipt of infected blood or blood products virtually guarantees that the recipient will contract HIV infection.

Today the possibility of contracting HIV through contaminated blood is virtually nil (in the United States). The virus is extremely fragile and can be killed by heating or cooling.[7] Blood tests can screen out any infected blood and that blood can be destroyed. One cannot be 100 percent certain, however, and it is recommended that, in cases of elective surgery, that one donates his or her own blood prior to the procedure. In a medical emergency one might consider whether it is better to risk immediate death or risk a less than 1 percent chance of HIV infection.

The above groups are those to be considered at potentially high risk for HIV/AIDS. However, health professionals should be aware of others that may not appear to be at high risk but certainly must be considered.

Blacks and Hispanics currently comprise 18 percent of the U.S. population. However, these two groups comprise almost 40 percent of all AIDS cases to date.[4] These figures do not account for those who are or may be HIV-positive. Although the virus is contracted by intimate contact of one kind or another, these groups are disproportionately effected.

The incidence of pediatric AIDS is quickly growing. Although there are fewer cases of transfusion AIDS, there remains a growing number of children born to mothers who are HIV positive. The current number of pediatric AIDS cases is approximately 2,200—with the vast majority being black and Hispanic.[4] Recent estimates indicate that the number of pediatric AIDS cases will reach as high as 10,000 to 20,000 by 1991.

Teenagers, regardless of their race, sexual preference or socioeconomic status, are a group who are at extremely high risk of HIV infection, as well as other diseases. As of April 1990, there were 500 documented cases of AIDS in persons between the ages of 13 to 19.[4] Researchers estimate that one in every 500 college students is HIV-positive.[8] The teenage years are a time of rebellion— breaking away from one's parents in order to establish autonomy. In this process, a great deal of experimentation with sex and drugs may occur. These activities are the very ones that put this group at risk. A recent survey[9] indicated that by age 17, 50 percent of all teenagers have been sexually active. Of this group, 53 percent of the males reported that they did not use a condom during intercourse and 16 percent of the females indicated that they had engaged in sexual intercourse with four or more separate partners. These figures are and should be alarming. When one considers that one out of every seven teenagers has had some type of sexually transmitted disease (STD) and there continues to be 1.2 million teenage pregnancies per year, it is obvious that the risk of HIV infection in this group is quite high.

Other groups, including the mentally retarded, emotionally disturbed, psychiatric patients, the homeless, the sexually abused and runaways should also be considered to be at high risk for HIV/AIDS, for they are all capable of sexual activity, IV drug use and contact with infected body fluids. In short, anyone is at risk and therefore, any treatment facility may encounter an individual with HIV/AIDS.

Health Care Professionals and Occupational Exposure

Perhaps the most common fear of and most frequently asked question by health professionals, concerns occupational exposure to HIV. Many are afraid to work with persons with HIV/AIDS for fear that they might contract the virus. The media occasionally relays stories of a physician or nurse who has been exposed to HIV infection through an accidental needle stick or by being splashed with a patient's blood. These incidents, while being undeniably tragic, are rare and, in many cases, resulted from improper procedure in dealing with blood and body fluids and the disposal of contaminated needles. Certain members of the health field are at higher risk for occupational exposure than are others: physicians, particularly dentists and surgeons, nurses and housekeeping personnel are frequently exposed to puncture wounds from needles and bone fragments. Others, including occupational therapists, are at less of a risk but should follow proper precautions (see Appendices B and C) when dealing with blood and body fluids to prevent exposure to, not only HIV, but to other diseases as well. These precautions should be followed with all patients regardless of their diagnosis.

It should be made clear that although HIV infection is on the rise, it is a difficult virus to contract. If one engages in safe sex techniques and does not share contaminated needles or receive contaminated blood, the possibility of contracting HIV infection is virtually nil. Casual contact is not a mode of transmitting HIV. Casual contact includes touching, hugging, shaking hands, transferring patients, eating food that is prepared and/or served by an infected individual, or sharing toothbrushes or eating utensils (this practice is not advised, however, as other diseases can be transmitted in this manner). Coughing and sneezing cannot transfer HIV, although many other common viruses are obviously spread in this manner.

Many people are concerned about the transmission of HIV by way of mosquito bites. This also is not a possible route. The average mosquito can consume and digest only one blood meal per day. When one considers that HIV is an extremely delicate virus and is easily killed by both environmental and chemical factors, that is, temperature and digestive enzymes, one can be assured that the possibility if HIV inoculation is highly unlikely. If HIV could be transmitted in a casual manner, the incidence of the disease would be hundreds of times higher than the current figures indicate.

Stages of HIV Infection

Once the virus has been introduced into the body and has established itself within its host cells, the infected individual will enter the first of four main classifications and possibly progress through the remaining three. These groups are: HIV-positive, asymptomatic, PGL, ARC, and the final stage of AIDS.

The individual who is HIV-positive, asymptomatic has been exposed to the virus and has developed antibodies to it. However, there may be no overt symptoms of disease and, unless the individual has been tested, they may be unaware of their condition. In a way, this can be the most dangerous stage of the disease in terms of unknowingly passing the virus to others through unprotected sex or by the sharing of needles.

With PGL, the individual will experience swollen glands and perhaps a low-grade fever for a period of three months or longer. During this stage, the individual may not feel completely well but may not suspect anything out of the ordinary and, therefore, may not seek treatment.

With ARC the individual is clearly ill and it is in this stage that many are diagnosed with HIV infection. ARC is manifested by unexplained weight loss, persistent fever, oral thrush, chronic diarrhea and soaking night sweats. Many individuals have reported that, due to the profuse sweating, they had to change their sheets as many as three to four times a night. Often the demarcation between ARC and AIDS is vague and the clinical usefulness of the ARC classification is questionable.[10]

The final stage of HIV disease is AIDS. The hallmarks of AIDS are a T-cell count of less than 400 cells/mm^3 (a normal T-cell count is approximately 1,600 cell/mm^3), the presence of certain opportunistic infections, specifically PCP and KS, HIV encephalopathy, and HIV wasting syndrome. It is in this stage that the body is plagued by the host of opportunistic infections (Appendix D) which are associated with AIDS and other conditions in which the immune system is severely compromised. Death in these individuals occurs not from HIV itself, but rather the opportunistic diseases (particularly PCP) or from complications such as renal failure and cardiac arrest. It should be noted that while most deaths occur in AIDS, it is possible that an infected individual can die from complications in any of the other stages as well. Figure 12-1 outlines the current stages of HIV infection according to the CDC.

Of those individuals who have been exposed to HIV, it has been estimated that 20 percent remain positive, asymptomatic; 20 to 30 percent develop PGL; 20 percent develop ARC; and 30 percent progress to full-spectrum AIDS.[11]. Due to the relative newness of the disease process, it is difficult to predict if all infected individuals will progress to full-spectrum AIDS. There are many factors to be considered in the progression of the disease among individuals: genetic predisposition, post-morbid lifestyle, the ability to deal with stress, the presence of other disease processes and perhaps the individual's overall personality. It is also difficult, at this time, to determine how effective the administration of drugs such as AZT and DDI is in the retarding of the disease process.

Tests for HIV Infection

Currently, there are only two serologic assays on the market that can be used to detect the presence of antibodies to HIV: the enzyme linked immunoabsorbent assay (ELISA) and the Western blot. It is important to note that neither of these tests will detect the actual presence of HIV in the blood. Therefore, if an individual has been infected and no antibodies have been formed at the time of the test, the results will probably be negative. The ELISA is the more common of the two and a positive result will be confirmed by the longer and more expensive Western blot. A newer serologic test, the single-use diagnostic system (SUDS), has been recently introduced for a more rapid analysis of a given blood sample. Although the SUDS offers results in as little as 15 minutes, there are concerns that the general employment of this test will compromise confidentiality and make the HIV-positive individual vulnerable to bias.

One test, the polymerized chain reaction (PCR), is used to test for the presence of HIV. The PCR is usually used to determine if HIV DNA is an inherent part of fetal cells or if it is part of the mother's antibodies. It can also be used to confirm HIV infection who may be at high risk of infection but who test negative by other test methods.

The testing of individuals for HIV antibodies has become both a legal and emotional issue. Many persons who are known to be HIV-positive have lost their jobs, been denied health insurance, and been ostracized from society. For these and other reasons, many people who may be at risk for HIV choose not to be tested to preserve their lives and their livelihoods. Testing procedures should not be taken lightly and should always include both pre- and post-test counseling. Early testing is extremely important if treatment is

Group I	Acute infection (mononucleosis syndrome, aseptic meningitis—HIV antibody negative/positive)
Group II	Asymptomatic infection (+HIV, subclassify by laboratory abnormalities)
Group III	Persistent generalized lymphodenopathy (+HIV)
Group IV	Other diseases

	Subgroup A	Constitutional disease (weight loss, fever)
	Subgroup B	Neurologic disease (dementia, neuropathy, myelopathy)
	Subgroup C	Secondary infectious diseases

	Category C-1	Specified secondary infectious diseases (PCP, MAI, CMV, cryptococcosis, cryptosporidiosis, CNS toxoplasmosis, chronic or diss. HSV)
	Category C-2	Other specified secondary infectious diseases (tuberculosis, oral candiasis, diss., variella zoster virus (VZV), nocardiosis)

	Subgroup D	Secondary cancers (Kaposi's sarcoma, lymphoma, immunoblastic sarcoma)
	Subgroup E	Other conditions (chronic lymphoid interstitial pneumonia)

Figure 12-1. CDC classification system for HIV Infection. *Source: Centers for Disease Control.*

to be rendered in a timely fashion. Although there is currently no cure for AIDS, early intervention can retard the progress of the disease and prevent or reduce many of the unpleasant opportunistic infections that accompany it.

Neurologic Sequelae of HIV Infection

The effects of HIV infection on the human body extend beyond the familiar Kaposi's lesions and PCP episodes, reaching and undermining both the CNS and peripheral nervous system with a Pandora's box of neuropathology. These neurologic problems may occur directly from HIV infection itself, neoplasms and secondary neurologic infections, or reactions to medications used in the patient's treatment.[12] AIDS produces clinical neurologic complications in about 40 percent of patients, and about 10 percent initially have with neurologic complications.[13] The occupational therapist working with these individuals should be aware of the scope of neurologic involvement in persons with AIDS to render effective treatment. While it is not always critical to obtain a specific differential diagnosis in all cases, the therapist should be aware of the broad spectrum of clinical signs and symptoms that may be present. The standard assessments, evaluations and basic treatment principles that are part of the therapist's knowledge base are useful, appropriate and applicable in the treatment of these individuals.[12]

Primary HIV Infection

As we have already stated, HIV is attracted to cells that contain CD4 as part of their outer membrane, including the support cells, or neuroglia, of the CNS. Because HIV is able to cross the blood-brain barrier, the CNS is quite vulnerable to direct HIV infection in addition to secondary infections.

The result of CNS HIV infection is manifested in a form of dementia which has come to be known as AIDS dementia complex (ADC), HIV encephalopathy, or subacute encephalitis. This syndrome causes a variety of clinical symptoms including poor concentration, decreased memory, psychomotor retardation and social withdrawal. Later manifestations may include confusion, disorientation, seizures, ataxia and coma. The patient frequently will present with an abnormal mental status examination as well as frontal release signs.[14]

Patients with ADC often require constant supervision to prevent them from doing harm to themselves out of forgetfulness or impaired judgment, much like the patient with Alzheimer's disease. Similarly, these individuals, particularly those in the mild to moderate stages, may experience great difficulty in performing daily living skills such as bathing, dressing and meal preparation and will require a great deal of, if not total, assistance with these activities.[15] Individuals in the early stages may benefit from written instructions and reminders, prepoured medication doses, and rote training. For those in the later stages, therapeutic intervention might better be directed toward helping the caregiver to cope, rather than toward the patient directly.

Secondary Neurologic Diseases

In lieu of, or in addition to, the effects of primary HIV infection of the CNS, the patient may experience one or more secondary neurologic infections that frequently accompany advanced HIV disease. These infections can effect virtually any level of the neuraxis and produce a variety of clinical symptoms, most of which should be familiar to the practicing therapist. The therapist should not be surprised to see symptoms such as sensory deficits such as decreased proprioception and tactile sensation, as well as causalgia which can result from dorsal column and medial lemniscus involvement. Additionally, about 10 to 15 percent of AIDS patients develop CMV retinitis as the result of direct infection of the retina by CMV which often results in blindness.[16]

Pyramidal and extrapyramidal signs are also encountered as descending motor paths become involved. These symptoms which include ataxia, hypotonia, hypertonia, and movement disorders such as ballistic movements, result from both direct infection of specific structures such as the basal ganglia[17] or space-occupying lesions within the brain and spinal cord. Many patients present with hemiplegia or quadriplegia as a result of these infections and may be treated as would a patient with a stroke or spinal cord injury. However, it is possible that these individuals will develop further neurologic signs as other structures within the CNS or PNS become involved. For example, an individual who initially presents with left-sided spastic hemiparesis could suddenly develop an LUE flaccid paralysis as the result of a lesion at the brachial plexus. The addition of further insults and resulting loss of progress and function can be very disconcerting to the patient, the caregiver and the therapist. For this reason it is important

Neurologic Disorders	Clinical Manifestations
Opportunistic Infections	
Toxoplasma gondii	Cerebral mass lesions (i.e., encephalopathy and focal neurologic deficits)
Cryptococcal meningitis	Headache, encephalopathy, cranial neuropathy
Aseptic meningitis	Headache,frequent recurrence
Progressive multifocal leukoencephalopathy	Dementia, blindness, ataxia, hemiparesis
Miscellaneous viral encephalitis (CMV, herpes simplex)	Encephalopathy, headaches, seizures, focal deficits, rarely as myelopathy
Miscellaneous nonviral infections (mycobacteria, *treponema allidum*, candida)	Variable (depending on the organism, may present as mass lesions, meningitis, or encephalitis)
Miscellaneous	
AIDS dementia complex	Dementia
Vacuolar myelopathy	Spasticity, parathesias, paraparesis
Primary CNS lymphoma	Similiar to other cerebral mass lesions
Systemic lymphoma	Spinal cord compression, cranial neuropathy, and radiculopathy
Kaposi's sarcoma	Cerebral mass lesions
Stroke	Similiar to stroke in the general population

Figure 12-2. Clinical manifestations of common central nervous system disorders in HIV-infected patients. *Adapted from So, Y. (1989). Neurologic manifestations of AIDS. AIDS Clinical Care, 1(5):38. Reprinted by permission of the New England Journal of Medicine.*

that the therapist possess a fundamental knowledge of the possible neurologic implications to initiate and alter an effective treatment program as necessary. Figures 12-2 and 12-3 list some of the common infections of the CNS and peripheral nervous system and the clinical manifestations they produce.

Children who become infected prenatally frequently exhibit neurologic involvement which can present clinical signs similar to those of cerebral palsy. Many may present with fetal AIDS syndrome[18] which includes growth failure and craniofacial abnormalities, including microcephaly in addition to sensorimotor disorders.

Due to the potential for neurologic involvement and the limitless possibilities of clinical signs associated with HIV infection, the therapist working with this population should be aware that many patients exhibit symptoms that are both physical and psychiatric. To be sure, those with only overt physical symptoms may suffer from depression over their situation. Similarly, a patient who initially

Neurologic Disorders	Clinical Manifestations
Neuropathies	
Distal symmetric polyneuropathy	Distal bilateral paresthesis, pain, loss of reflex
Demyelinating neuropathy	Weakness, sensory loss, loss of reflex
Mononeuropathy multiplex	Asymmetric weakness and sensory loss
Lumbosacral polyradiculopathy	Leg weakness and sensory loss, reflex loss, loss of sphincter control
Myopathies	
Myositis (some but not all are associated with AZT)	Symmetric proximal weakness in upper and lower extremities

Figure 12-3. Peripheral nervous system complications of HIV infection. *Adapted from So, Y. (1989). Neurologic manifestations of AIDS. AIDS Clinical Care, 1(5):39. Reprinted by permission of the New England Journal of Medicine.*

presents with dementia may develop physical involvement with the onset of secondary infections. The therapist must be cognizant of these changes and maintain good communication with the rest of the health care team in order to meet the ever changing needs of the patient.

Universal Precautions

One of the greatest fears among health care personnel is that of contracting AIDS during the performance of their assigned duties. As we have already pointed out, it is extremely difficult to contract HIV infection except for direct contact with infected body fluids. However, certain precautions should be taken to prevent possible exposure to the virus (see Appendices B and C). These precautions serve a dual function in that they reduce the health professional's risk of infection from the patient and also reduce the patient's risk of infection from the health-care provider. Infections transmitted from person to person or objects to person within a health-care facility are known as nosocomial infections. In terms of the patient with HIV/AIDS, the patient is actually at a greater risk of contracting a pathogen from the staff, than the staff is of contracting HIV from the patient. Therefore, when one employs various precautions to prevent infection, an explanation to the patient will demonstrate your concern for his health and facilitate the therapeutic relationship.

It is paramount that universal precautions be employed with **all** patients, not just those with known HIV infection. It is not possible to tell if someone is HIV positive just by looking at them or other subjective measurements. Conversely, there are a multitude of bacteria and viruses that are much more easily transmitted by more casual means such as touching: hepatitis, types A and B, staphylococcal infections, influenza and the common cold are but a few examples. These pathogens can affect anyone under normal conditions, and those individuals with compromised immune functions are particularly vulnerable. By employing proper universal precautions with all patients, the spread of pathogens from person to person can be reduced significantly.

Handwashing

As is often the case, the most efficient and effective means of accomplishing a goal is frequently the simplest one. Such is the case of infection control. By far, the most efficient method of disease prevention in professional practice, as well as in daily life, is the washing of one's hands. The intact skin is the body's first line of defense in the prevention of disease. At the same time it is a breeding ground for millions of indiscernible bacteria and viruses which can easily be transmitted from person to person through simple touch. By regularly washing one's hands, the transmission process can be interrupted. Although almost everyone washes his hands on a regular basis before eating or after using the toilet, the process is often taken for granted and hands are not washed as frequently as they should be. Hands must be washed at the following times:

1. Before starting work
2. Before and after treating individual patients
3. Before applying and after removing gloves
4. During performance of normal duties
5. Before and after the handling of food
6. After personal use of the toilet or toileting of a patient
7. After sneezing, coughing or contact with oral and nasal areas
8. Before eating or preparing food
9. Prior to leaving the rooms of patients on isolation or precautions
10. On completion of duty

Procedure for Proper Handwashing. Before washing your hands, you must have the following equipment: soap or detergent (preferably a liquid type, as bar type soap can breed bacteria), paper towels or forced air dryer, a sink with mixed hot and cold faucets, a waste container and hand lotion.

1. Remove rings, bracelets and watch
2. Inspect skin and nails for dryness, cracking, hangnails and cuts/abrasions. Fingernails should be short, smooth and free of chipped nail polish
3. Turn on faucets and maintain a comfortably warm water temperature. Avoid touching the sink with hands
4. Hold hands and wrists parallel to the floor or lower than elbows throughout the procedure
5. Add soap or detergent to hands
6. Rub palms together to produce lather
7. Using one lathered hand to wash the other, grasp one wrist and cleanse it by using friction to apply lather around it. Next apply lather with friction over the dorsum of the hand. Proceed to clean the dorsum of the fingers with the fingers flexed to expose creases at knuckles

8. Using friction, clean the lateral aspects of fingers and hands by interdigitation; rub right thumb over left and then left over right
9. Clean under fingernails with fingernail of the other hand or nail brush
10. Rinse under nails, then over wrists and hands using friction to remove suds
11. Repeat steps four through ten
12. Pat hands and wrists with paper towel to absorb excess water. Use a second towel to complete drying. Hands should be thoroughly dried to prevent chapping of skin which can allow pathogens to gain entry into the body
13. Use the dry side of second towel or third towel to turn off faucets (faucets are contaminated)
14. Dispose of towels properly
15. Apply hand lotion to maintain skin integrity

Although it is impossible to completely prevent contamination, except under the most sterile of conditions, by following the above guidelines, the therapist can prevent infection from spreading to himself, inanimate objects, other staff and patients. To further facilitate this process the therapist should be diligent in instructing others of the importance of proper handwashing techniques. This should include the patient, family members and significant others, other professional staff, home health or personal care aides, and housekeeping personnel. Again, these procedures should be followed with all patients and particularly when the patient is known to have a compromised immune system.

Use of Protective Barriers

There are instances when handwashing alone is insufficient such as when the patient is in isolation or when one is exposed to blood and body fluids. In these instances, protective barriers should be employed. These barriers can include band-aids, finger cots, gloves, masks, gowns and protective face wear and eye wear. When working with a patient with HIV disease gloves, masks, gowns and eye wear may be necessary at one time or another but not always. The practicing therapist must be vigilant about monitoring the integrity of his/her own skin integrity as well as that of the patient; particularly the skin of the hands. Any open wounds, including hangnails, broken cuticles, paper cuts and open, weeping dermatitis should be properly covered. In many instances, a band-aid or finger cot should provide sufficient protection for both the therapist and the patient. The wound should be thoroughly cleansed and dressed before treatment begins.

Gloves should be used when one comes into direct contact with blood and/or body fluids. This situation may arise frequently during the course of occupational therapy intervention, regardless of the setting, and a supply of gloves should always be available for use. These situations may include cleaning up urine, fecal matter or vomitus, dressing an open, bleeding wound, or toileting a patient. If one is treating a hand injury with an open wound from trauma or surgery, gloves should also be worn. When handling body fluids, it is not always possible to know if your hands have minute cuts and therefore gloves should be used to prevent infection. Again, these precautions are not specific to HIV only. Virtually any organism can be contracted in this manner and the therapist should be more concerned with pathogens such as hepatitis rather than with HIV. Any number of diseases can be contracted from any patient at any time.

Masks and gowns are often necessary if the patient is in some form of isolation (Figure 12-4). In these cases, the patient's chart and room indicate what type of precautions are necessary to prevent infection. If the patient is coughing up sputum, a mask is recommended if the therapist is working within three feet of the patient's face. It should be reiterated that HIV cannot be spread/contracted in an aerosol manner. However, many other infections can be and the therapist should consider this and take appropriate precautions. This is good advice for working with any patient, not only those with HIV/AIDS. In instances when the therapist feels that he might be at risk for spreading a cold or virus to a patient, a mask should be used during treatment—if treatment is not deferred. The difficulty in this situation is that when one is in the contagious stages of an illness, symptoms are often not present and do not appear until after the person has inadvertently infected others.

Protective face wear and eye wear is indicated only in situations where there is the possibility being splashed in the face with blood or body fluids. It seems unlikely that an occupational therapist would be in a situation of this nature and therefore, these precautions are usually not indicated in the course of treatment.

Should one come into contact with blood or other body fluids known to transmit HIV and no barriers are utilized, for example, if a patient cut himself while performing a woodworking activity and the therapist were splashed with blood, the body part that was struck by the blood should be washed immediately with a detergent and the skin integrity inspected. Detergent will break down the lipid outer membrane of HIV (and other viruses) and destroy it, preventing inoculation. A mild (10 percent) chlorine solution will also effectively kill the virus. When dressing the patient's wound and cleaning up any spilled blood, gloves should be worn and the area thoroughly cleaned and disinfected.

Infection Control in Occupational Therapy Practice

Regardless of what area of practice one is active in, it is of utmost importance to follow stringent infection control policy and procedure. When any number of patients is treated in an occupational therapy clinic, there is an increased possibility for contaminants to be spread from one individual or another either by direct contact or by contact with contaminated objects (fomites). Regular cleaning and disinfection can reduce the incidence of disease transmission and should be employed as part of departmental policy and procedure. The clinic should be well stocked with a regular supply of clean linens, paper towels, soap and/or detergent, disinfectant and a bucket and mop. A well-stocked first aid kit should also be available, as well as an adequate supply of latex gloves.

Common areas such as work tables, mats, bathrooms and kitchens should be cleaned before and after each use. Mats and beds should be covered with a fresh sheet before each patient uses them. Therapeutic equipment such as balls, cones, wedges and bolsters, standing frames and exercise equipment should be cleaned before and after use. Similarly, evaluation equipment such as goniometers, dynamometers and anesthesiometers should also be disinfected before and after each use.

Common Diseases that Require Isolation

Type of Isolation	Private Room	Gown	Gloves	Mask	Linen Precautions	Dish
Strict Isolation Smallpox, vaccinia, pneumonic plague, inhalation anthrax, varicella, disseminated herpes zoster, diptheria, rabies, burns infected with *Staphylococcus aureus* and group A streptococci	X	X	X	X	X	X
Modified strict isolation Staphyloccoccal and streptococcal pneumonia; all patients with copious sputum containing large numbers of coagulase-positive staphylococci or group A beta-hemolytic streptococci	X	+	+	X	X	X
Respiratory isolation Pulmonary tuberculosis, rubeola, mumps, rubella, pertussis, meningococcal meningitis,meningococcemia, viral hepatitis An accompanied by copious respiratory secretions which require suctioning.	X	–	–	X	–	–

Figure 12-4. Isolation Precautions. CDC classification system for HIV infection. *Adapted from Isolation Techniques for Use in Hospitals, U.S. Public Health Service Publication stock #017-023-00094-2. Washington, DC: Government Printing Office, Superintendent of Documents.*

Common Diseases that Require Isolation

Type of Isolation	Private Room	Gown	Gloves	Mask	Linen Precautions	Dish
Protective (reverse) isolation Agranulocytosis, lymphoma, immunosuppressant therapy, extensive noninfected burns; severe noninfected eczematous dermatitis	X	+	+	X	–	–
Enteric precautions Hepatitis A, cholera, salmonellosis, shigellosis, nonbacterial gastroenteritis, staphyococcal enterocolitis	D	X	X	–	X	X
Wound and skin precautions All wound and skin infections that can adequately contain drainage	X	+	+	+	X	–
Blood precautions Type B hepatitis, type non-A, non-B hepatitis, HIV, arthropod-borne viral fever (dengue)	X	–	X	–	+	+

Secretion precautions
Infected ischemic ulcers, decubitus ulcers, stitch abscesses, infected wounds in which drainage is minimal, gas, gangrene, impetigo

Double-bag soiled dressings and equipment. Use meticulous handwashing technique.

KEY
 X always necessary
 + = necessary only in direct contact with patient, secretions or contaminateed articles.
 D = desirable but optional
 – = unnecessary

Figure 12-4. Continued.

Eating utensils should be thoroughly cleaned, preferably in a dishwasher. If a dishwasher is not available these items should be washed in hot soapy water, rinsed in hot water, and allowed to air dry. Patients should not share eating utensils or other personal items such as toothbrushes, combs or hair brushes and the like. Spills of any kind, particularly urine (not a source of HIV transmission), feces or blood should be cleaned up immediately and the area disinfected. When cleaning body fluids of any kind, especially blood, gloves should always be worn and hands washed afterward.

Patients should be encouraged to maintain good personal hygiene and to wash their hands at the beginning and end of therapy sessions.

Housekeeping should clean the clinic thoroughly on a daily basis and should be called to perform emergency cleanups during the course of the workday.

Occupational Therapy Intervention with the HIV/AIDS Patient

In general, the goals of occupational therapy intervention with the AIDS patient will be the same as for any other patient whom one might encounter in everyday practice: that is, maximizing the patient's independence in daily living skills and effective interaction with the environment. Certainly, many of the symptoms and problem areas encountered by these individuals mimic other diseases and disabilities which the occupational therapist is already familiar with. There are, however, certain aspects of treatment that are important to stress in terms of working with this population which can help the patient to maintain a reasonable quality of life. These areas are addressed according to the uniform terminology as outlined by the American Occupational Therapy Association.[19] The following information does not cover all aspects of the uniform terminology but rather those areas in need of special consideration for the patient with HIV/AIDS.

Self-Care Role Performance Components

Self care skills are those that are required for daily living tasks and performance of daily personal care. They include grooming and hygiene, feeding and eating, dressing, functional mobility and object manipulation.[19]

Grooming and Hygiene. Grooming and hygiene refers to the skill and performance of personal health needs, such as bathing, toileting, hair care, shaving and applying make-up.[19] This is perhaps one of the most important areas of occupational therapy intervention with the patient with HIV/AIDS. Due to the body's inability to fight off infections, it is important that the patient maintain proper and regular hygiene practices to this end. Daily bathing and regular washing of hands throughout the day can reduce the possibility of undue infections caused by pathogens which are harbored in the skin and hair. The patient should always wash his hands after using the bathroom or contact with his own body fluids such as semen, mucus or blood, as well as before preparing and eating foods.[21] By being clean and well groomed, the patient's morale will also be improved which can lead to feelings of self-confidence and improved self-esteem. This is important to all patients but it is of particular importance to those with AIDS as a reduced sense of self-esteem increases the risk of illness.[20] The patient should also be made aware of the importance of caring for breaks in the skin and to inspect the skin for any abnormalities such as fungal infections, KS lesions, sebborhea, psoriasis or other skin problems. If the patient wears pierced earrings he should be instructed to thoroughly clean and disinfect the earring(s) and ear lobes before inserting the earrings to reduce the possibility of infection. Similarly, if the patient wears contact lenses, these should be cleaned and disinfected on a daily basis to prevent the possibility of eye infections (there is no evidence that persons with HIV/AIDS have a higher incidence of eye infections from contact lenses. This precaution is designed to reduce the possibility of an unnecessary problem). If the patient wears any type of orthotic device, such as a hand splint, this device should also be cleaned and disinfected on a daily basis to prevent the buildup of bacteria on the surfaces.

Feeding and Eating. Feeding/eating refers to the skill and performance of sequentially feeding oneself, including sucking, chewing, swallowing, and using appropriate utensils.[19] Many patients may have difficulty bringing food to their mouths due to paralysis, weakness, movement disorders or sensory deficits. Others may experience dysphagia brought about by cranial nerve involvement or by oral thrush which is caused by Candida infection.

Dressing. Dressing refers to the skill and performance of choosing appropriate clothing, dressing oneself in a sequential fashion, including fastening and adjusting clothing.[19] Problems in this area can result from sensory and/or motor involvement, as well as dementia. By allowing the patient to dress on a daily basis, the sick role or patient role can be replaced by the person role by empowering the individual.

Functional Mobility. Functional mobility refers to the skill and performance in moving oneself from one position or place to another. It includes skills necessary for activities such as bed mobility, wheelchair mobility, transfers (bed, car, tub, toilet, chair) and functional mobility with or without assistive devices. It also includes the use of public and private travel systems, such as driving one's own automobile or using public transportation.[19] Movement is an important part of maintaining one's autonomy and one's health. By engaging in these activities, many secondary conditions such as upper respiratory and urinary tract infections, decubiti and contractures, all of which can result from prolonged immobility, can be reduced or prevented.

Object Manipulation. Object manipulation refers to the skill and performance in handling large and small common objects, such as calculators, keys, money, light switches, doorknobs and packages.[19] Problems here can result from sensorimotor impairments as well as dementia.

Work Role Performance Components

Work refers to the skill and performance in participating in socially purposeful and productive activities. These activities take place in the home, employment setting, school and community. They include, but are not limited to, homemaking/home management, child care/parenting and employment preparation.[19] We will discuss only home management skills with the emphasis on areas that will be of particular importance to the patient with HIV/AIDS and their caregivers.

Homemaking and Home Management. Homemaking refers to the skill and performance in tasks such as meal planning, meal preparation and clean up, laundry, cleaning, household chores, minor household repairs, shopping, budgeting and use of household safety principles.[19] For the patient with HIV/AIDS, independent living and the management of the home can often be difficult and frequently overwhelming. There are certain tasks that must be performed adequately to reduce the possibility of unwanted infection that may result from improper housekeeping skills.

In general, the living area should be kept as clean and uncluttered as possible to avoid accidental falls. Two areas of particular importance are the bathroom and the kitchen. In addition to being the two rooms in that accidents occur most frequently, they are, by virtue of their utility, the rooms that can serve as exceptional breeding grounds for pathogens.

The bathroom should be cleaned on a daily basis. Chlorinated cleansers should be used and/or a 1:10 solution of bleach and water. The toilet and/or commode, the sink, and the bathtub are of particular importance. Other items such as grab bars and tub benches should also be thoroughly cleaned and disinfected. If the patient will be performing these tasks, they should be encouraged to wear a pair of rubber gloves to avoid contact with pathogens. The gloves should be disinfected prior to removal. A commercial disinfectant such as Lysol will help to reduce contamination as well. The patient and/or caregiver should be instructed to clean up any and all spills on the floor to prevent accidental falls.

The kitchen should also be cleaned and disinfected on a daily basis, with special attention paid to the sink and food preparation areas. The kitchen floor should be mopped at least once a week and mop water should not be poured down the sink where food is prepared.[21] Sponges that are used to clean the bathroom, body fluids and floor spills should not be used to wash dishes or clean food preparation areas. Sponges and mops can be disinfected with 1:10 bleach for five minutes (longer periods of time may disintegrate the sponge).[21] The refrigerator should be cleaned on a weekly basis and any spoiled food items should be discarded. All crumbs and food scraps should be properly disposed of to avoid attracting disease-carrying insects such as cockroaches.

Any foods that will be eaten by the patient should be thoroughly cooked to kill any parasites or other organisms that could cause gastrointestinal or other systemic problems. Organically grown foods should be avoided as they may have been fertilized with human or animal waste. Raw foods such as sushi, clams and raw eggs should also be avoided as they are known to carry parasites and diseases such as hepatitis A, which can be problematic for a healthy individual and potentially lethal to those with a depleted immune response. Any and all dairy products which the patient will eat should be pasteurized.[22] Dishes used to hold raw or uncooked foods such as meat or vegetables should not be used to hold the same food items after cooking unless they have been washed with hot, soapy water. Bacteria that are present on these foods before cooking may linger on the vessel and re-contaminate the food even though the food has been properly prepared.

Dishes and eating utensils should be washed thoroughly after each use. These items should be washed in a dishwasher for optimal results. If no dishwasher is available, eating utensils should be washed in hot, soapy water, rinsed in hot water and rack dried (dish towels can harbor germs). Due to the necessity of using hot water, insulated rubber gloves are highly recommended for this task, especially for patients who have sensory impairments. Dishwater should be changed for each washing. It should not be allowed to sit as it can serve as a breeding ground for bacteria.

Trash should be disposed of immediately and properly. Plastic trash bags should be used and securely sealed before transporting. The patient should wear gloves when handling the trash and wash their hands after removing the gloves. If the patient requires any injectable medications such as insulin, used needles should **never** be disposed of with the regular trash. These needles should be disposed of in special "sharps" containers that can be obtained through visiting nurse or similar programs. The patient should be made aware that others can be put at risk if needles are not disposed of properly.

Laundry should be done on a regular basis using hot soapy water and bleach. Bed linens and clothes soiled with feces and body fluids should be washed separately. If possible, bed linens should be changed on a daily basis.

If the patient has any pets, he must be aware of certain considerations to prevent possible infection. All pets should be carefully examined by a veterinarian for the presence of any diseases that might be passed onto the patient. Pets should be kept in the house to prevent the possibility of them picking up diseases from other animals and the outdoor environment. Stray animals should be avoided as pets, unless they are examined by the vet prior to admission to the home. The patient should exercise extreme caution when changing litter boxes (a source of toxoplasmosis and psittacosis),[21] bird cages (cryptococcus), turtle dishes (salmonella), and even fish bowls (mycobacterium).[21] If the patient must perform these tasks, gloves and masks should be worn and hands washed immediately afterward. Litter boxes, in particular, should be changed on a daily basis as it takes *Toxoplasma gondii* approximately 48 hours to proliferate within the stools. Furthermore, cat scratches can result in bacillary epithelioid angiomatosis (BEA)[23] and cat owners should be warned to avoid cat scratches.

It is important for the patient to realize that any waste product can harbor opportunistic infections and extreme care should be exercised when performing such tasks.

Although pet wastes pose potential threats to the PWA's health, pet ownership should not be discouraged. To be sure, pets can add a great deal to the individual's quality of life and many believe that pets can be beneficial to both the physical and psychological well-being of an ill individual. Studies have shown

that persons who have had heart attacks have a higher chance of survival if they
have pets waiting for them at home.[24] Similarly, patients in hospitals, including
psychiatric facilities, are reported to recover faster and are discharged sooner
when pets are around.[24]

It may often be difficult for many patients to handle the rigors of self care role
performance due to medical complications, decreased endurance or dementia.
If the therapist discerns that some or all aspects of self-care are unrealistic for the
patient to perform, treatment should then be directed at the caregiver, as they
are acting as the patient's agent in these tasks.

Psychological/Emotional Personal Role Performance Elements

Psychological/emotional daily living skills refer to the skill and performance
in developing one's self-concept and self-identity, coping with life situations, and
participating in one's organizational and community environment. They include, but are not limited to, self-concept and self-identity, situational coping,
cognitive and psychosocial components.[19] Although all of these components are
of extreme importance to the patient with HIV/AIDS, we will focus only on
situational coping, as this area can have a direct impact on the patient's health.

Situational coping refers to the skill and performance in handling stress and
dealing with problems and changes in a manner that is functional for self and
others. This includes, but is not limited to

- Setting goals, selecting, harmonizing, and managing activities of daily living to
  promote optimal performance
- Testing goals and perceptions against reality
- Perceiving changes and need for changes in self and environment
- Directing and redirecting energy to overcome problems
- Initiating, implementing, and following through on decisions
- Assuming responsibility for self and consequences of actions
- Interacting with others: dyadic and group[19]

Studies have shown that stress can exacerbate the symptoms of HIV/AIDS and
facilitate the disease process. The ability to cope with stress seems to be a factor
in who remains asymptomatic or undergoes mild illness and who gets the fully
developed disease.[25] It has been observed that in a group of HIV-positive men, all
of those who developed full-spectrum AIDS reported experiencing unresolved
stressful situations prior to the onset of the disease.[26] Furthermore, stress has
been found to increase tumor growth in laboratory animals[27] and probably in
humans as well. During examination periods, medical students have a decrease
in their blood levels of both interferons and natural killer cells, two active agents
in the immune system.[28] The effect of stress on immune function, although not
entirely understood, is thought to weaken the immune response by the release of
high amounts of adrenal hormones into the system.[29] The sympathetic nervous
system can also affect the immune system directly by its innervation of the thymus
gland, spleen and lymph nodes.[30] Other studies have demonstrated that by
reducing stress in patients with AIDS and other diseases, the disease process can
be governed to some degree, by bolstering the immune system.[31] Occupational
therapy intervention in this area can serve to be prophylactic in nature, rather

than tertiary, in terms of the disease process. By promoting independence and balance in daily life skills and thus empowering the patient, the occupational therapist can assist in reducing the stress response and replace it with a health response. The relaxation response can be facilitated with a variety of techniques including relaxation training, imaging, yoga, and biofeedback. Pain, which is common to many persons with AIDS, can prolong the stress response and in turn, stress can exacerbate the pain. This stress/pain cycle can be interrupted by relaxation techniques, as well as by massage and devices such as transcutaneous electrical nerve stimulators (TENS), which can allow the patient to gain increased function.[32] Many people attempt to alleviate stress by using alcohol, nicotine, and other substances to relax. The efficacy of this approach in a healthy individual is questionable at best. The use of these substances by a person with HIV/AIDS can be detrimental to their health in that many of these substances, particularly alcohol and tobacco, can weaken the immune system even further.[33] This information should be shared with the patient for him to make the decision to continue using them or not.

Nontraditional Roles for the Occupational Therapist

AIDS has caused everyone in the health-care community to reexamine their roles in the treatment of those who are afflicted with this disease; occupational therapists are and should be no different. There are many areas that must be addressed with the patient and their family and significant others concerning the disease. Education is paramount. It is unwise to assume that because someone has AIDS that they know everything or anything about it. It is the duty of all health care professionals to share whatever knowledge they can with their patients, their families and significant others.

The therapist should be prepared to instruct their patients in basic AIDS education, guidelines for safe sex, including the proper use and care of a condom, not to share needles and/or how to properly clean and disinfect needles if they are to be reused, special hygiene requirements for HIV-positive individuals, and be aware of and refer those in need of, the various AIDS organizations that are available in one's community. Certainly these are not traditional roles for the practicing therapist. However, it is necessary that they become part of the tradition of the practice.

It is likely that at some point in time, the HIV/AIDS patient will want to talk about the possibility or reality of his impending death. In these instances it is imperative that the occupational therapist be prepared to discuss the topic honestly and openly with the patient. To avoid the subject is to do a great injustice to the patient, who may have a real need to discuss his fears and concerns. Death is not a topic that many people, including health professionals, prefer to discuss. We are, after all, in the business of health and life. Death implies failure on our part—even if it is inevitable. We must realize that death is a part of life that must be acknowledged and accommodated.[34]

With the exception of those items outlined in this chapter, the role of the occupational therapist with the patient with HIV/AIDS is no different than

A. **Pre-AIDS**
1. Stress management
2. Education
3. Group intervention (activity/verbal combination)
4. Creative self-expression
5. Vocational/leisure assessment

B. **Phase 2: Early- to Mid- Stage Disease**
1. Standardized assessment (physical and psychosocial where applicable)
2. Therapeutic crafts
3. ADL intervention
4. Adaptive equipment
5. Cognitive remediation
6. Energy conservation/work simplification
7. Facilitation techniques such as PNF, NDT, etc.
8. Mobility training
9. Dysphagia intervention
10. Pain management
11. Self-ranging
12. Leisure/play activities
13. Orthotic fabrication
14. Discharge planning/home assessment
15. Consultation
16. Vocational planning/adaptation

C. **Phase 3: End-Stage Disease**
1. Discharge planning continued
2. Consultation (assistive devices, positioning, ADL, etc.)
3. Family, support system training
4. Reality orientation/sensory retraining
5. Creative self-expression/therapeutic crafts/leisure interests

Figure 12-5. Suggested Treatment Phases and Intervention Strategies. *Denton, R. (1987). AIDS: Guidelines for Occupational Therapy Intervention. American Journal of Occupational Therapy, 41(7):430. Used by permission.*

with that of any other patient population, and even those special considerations would benefit other populations. Denton[35] has outlined suggested occupational therapy treatment phases and intervention strategies for the patient with HIV/AIDS which can provide the therapist with an effective framework on which to base treatment (Figure 12-5). The goal of occupational therapy is to promote independence and health through a balance in the role performance areas of self-care, work and play/leisure. The *task* of occupational therapy is to prevent and reduce the incapacities resulting from illness.[36] The *job* of occupational therapy is to activate the residual adaptation forces within the patient.[36] The patient with AIDS is no different than any other patient with a serious or life-threatening illness. It is the stigma of the disease that makes them appear to be different. The occupational therapist can offer a unique and indispensable service to those with HIV/AIDS. While it is true that other professions such as medicine, nursing and nutrition can help these individuals to stay alive, the occupational therapist has the unique training and skills to help these individuals to *live*—regardless of their prognosis. Through the promotion of the individuals occupational roles, self-esteem, intrinsic motivation and physical abilities, occupational therapy can add significantly to the patient's quality of life experiences. In doing so, we can lend testimony to Reilly's[37] maxim: "Man, through the use of his hands, as they are energized by his mind and will, can influence the state of his own health."

References

1. Keeton, W.T. (1976). *Biological Science*, 3rd ed. New York: W.W. Norton, p. 919.

2. Langone, J. (1985). AIDS. *Discover*, (December): 28-53.

3. Centers for Disease Control (1987). Recommendations for the prevention of HIV transmission in healthcare settings. *Morbidity and Mortality Weekly Report*, 36:15-155.

4. U.S. Department of Health and Human Services (1990). *HIV/AIDS Surveillance*, (April):1-18.

5. Gay Mens Health Crisis (1987). *The Safer Condom Guide for Men and Women*. New York.

6. Marcil, W.M. (1988). Unpublished interviews with recovering substance abusers. February-March.

7. Merkens, M.J. and Cowell, S. (1988). *AIDS: Myths and Current Facts*. NY: Monroe County Department of Health, Rochester.

8. Biemiller, L. (1989). An average of 2 students in 1,000 found infected with AIDS-linked virus. *Chronicle of Higher Education*, (May): 1.

9. United States Department of Education (1988). *AIDS and the Education of Our Children: A Guide for Parents and Teachers*. Washington, DC: U.S. Government Printing Office, p. 5.

10. Clement, M. (1989). Patient care queries. *AIDS Clinical Care*, 1(7):62.

11. Rzepkowski, N. (1987). Medical Overview of AIDS. Staff Training Program. Albany, NY: AIDS Council of Northeastern New York.

12. Bonck, J. (1987). The neurological sequelae of AIDS: Treatment issues for occupational therapy. *Physical Disabilities Special Interest Section Newsletter*, 10(3):1, 6-7.

13. Simon, R.P., Aminoff, M.J. and Greenburg, D.H. (1989). *Clinical Neurology*. Norwalk, CT: Appleton & Lange, p. 29.

14. So, Y. (1989). Neurologic manifestations of AIDS. *AIDS Clinical Care*, 1(5):37-40.

15. Price, R.W. and Brew, B.J. (1988). The AIDS dementia complex. *Journal of Infectious Diseases*, 158(5):1079-1083.

16. O'Donnell, J.J. (1989). Treating cytomegalovirus retinitis. *AIDS Clinical Care*, 1(3):17-27.

17. Nath, A., Jankovic, J. and Creed-Pettigrew, L. (1987). Movement disorders and AIDS. *Neurology*, 37:37-41.

18. Marion, R.W., Wiznia, A.A., Hutcheon, R.G., et al. (1987). Fetal AIDS syndrome score. *American Journal of Disease in Children*, 141:429-431.

19. American Occupational Therapy Association (1979). *Uniform Terminology for Reporting Occupational Therapy Services*. Rockville, MD:AOTA.

20. Schmale, A.H. (1958). Relationship of separation and depression to disease. *Psychosomatic Medicine*, 20(4):259-274.

21. Lusby, G. and Schietinger, H. (1986). *Infection Control Precautions for People with AIDS Living in the Community*. Trenton, NJ: New Jersey State Department of Health.

22. Task Force on Nutrition Support in AIDS (1989). *Nutrition and AIDS: Taking Charge of Your Diet*. New York.

23. Clement, M. (1990). Patient care queries. *AIDS Clinical Care*, 2(4):29-36.

24. Messeni, P. (1984, June). Panel on Pets as Social Support. Meeting of the Pacific Division of the American Association for the Advancement of Science, San Francisco.

25. Bahnson, C.B. (1984, August). Psychological Aspects of AIDS. Symposium Summary of the Annual Meeting of the American Psychological Association, Toronto, Canada.

26. Fettner, A.G. and Check, W.A. (1984). *The Truth About AIDS*. New York:Holt, Rinehart and Winston.

27. Sklar, L.S. and Anisman, H (1981). Stress and cancer. *Psychological Bulletin*, 89:369-406.

28. Glaser, R., Rice, J., Speicher, C.E., et al. (1986). Stress depresses interferon production by leukocytes concommitant with a decrease in natural killer cell activity. *Behavioral Neuroscience*, 100:675-678.

29. Axelrod, J. and Reisine, T.D. (1984). Stress hormones: Their interaction and regulation. *Science*, 224:452-459.

30. Kalat, J.W. (1988). *Biological Psychology*, 3rd ed. Belmont, CA: Wadsworth Publishing Co., p. 328.

31. Goodkin, K., Glaser, R., Kiecolt-Glaser, J., et al. (1988). The link between attitude and the immune system in AIDS. Symposium Summary of the Annual Meeting of the American Association for the Advancement of Science, San Francisco.

32. Framroze, A. (1989). Coping with AIDS in the rehab environment. *REHAB Management*, 2(3):57-63.

33. Watson, R. and Darban, H. (1988). Alcohol and immunosuppression. *Clinical Immunology Newsletter*, 9(8):120-134.

34. Tigges, K.N. and Marcil, W.M. (1988). *Terminal and Life Threatening Illness: An Occupational Behavior Perspective*. Thorofare, NJ: Slack, p. 8.

35. Denton, R. (1987). AIDS: Guidelines for occupational therapy intervention. *American Journal of Occupational Therapy*, 41(7):430-431.

36. Reilly, M. (1969). The education process. *American Journal of Occupational Therapy*, 23:299-307.

37. Reilly, M. (1962). Occupational therapy can be one of the great ideas of twentieth century medicine. *American Journal of Occupational Therapy*, 16:1-9.

13 The Legal and Ethical Issues of AIDS

Mauro A. Montoya, Jr., Esq.

We hold these truths to be self-evident, that all men are created equal, that they are endowed by their creator with certain inalienable rights, that among these are life, liberty and the pursuit of happiness.
—The Declaration of Independence

Introduction

This chapter will explore some of the legal problems that persons with AIDS (PWAs) often face in the areas of government benefits, employment, insurance, landlord-tenant issues, and other areas of the law. A goal of the legal system, regarding PWAs, is to enhance the lives of all those infected, to the fullest extent possible, by ensuring that their rights are respected. The information provided in the following pages is meant to be general information and should *not* be used as absolute, in all instances. It is best to advise a patient to consult a lawyer as to specific questions or problems.

This chapter will also discuss some areas of concern to health-care providers: informed consent and liability of medical professionals in treating PWAs, as well as refusal to treat these patients.

Legal Issues For PWAS

There are three separate legal documents for PWAs to consider enacting. In terms of health care, the most important is the *durable medical power of attorney*. A legal power of attorney allows someone other than the patient, to transact that patient's business when the patient is unable to do so. A *last will* is also advisable, especially if children and/or property are involved. Finally, a *living will* will help the patient to decide to what extent medical treatment should be rendered in a terminal situation.

Powers of Attorney

A power of attorney allows the PWA to give someone else the legal ability to act on their behalf. The person appointed is called an *attorney-in-fact*. The attorney-in-fact does not have to be an actual attorney; merely a competent adult. There are different types of powers of attorney: A *specific power of attorney* allows someone to act on behalf of the patient for a specific purpose, such as receiving mail or writing checks. A *general power of attorney* allows the attorney-in-fact to do virtually everything that the patient would do, with the patient's signature. With a *valid power of attorney*, the attorney-in-fact can act as though he were the patient. Additionally, there are medical and legal powers of attorney.

A *medical power of attorney* lets the patient decide whom they want to make medical decisions for them rather than allowing the law to decide for them. Patients retain control over their medical treatment by using this document. Legally, people have the right to continue or refuse treatment as long as they are capable of making the decision. If they are unable to make such a decision, a family member has the legal right to make it for them, unless an attorney-in-fact has been designated. A valid power of attorney is especially important if the patient has a partner or friend whom he wants to make decisions for her or him. This is because the partner or friend has no legal status to make the decisions, unless they are legally married.

Health-care providers are often caught in a situation where the patient has not made a designation, but has a partner. The partner and the patient's family may each want to make decisions for the patient. In the event that a conflict should arise over this, the health-care provider may be caught in the middle, and vital decisions may be delayed. One way to alleviate this is for health-care providers to discuss, with the patient, whom they want their decisionmaker to be. The provider should document this in the patient's medical records. If the patient wants a person other than a family member, the health-care provider should encourage the patient to enact a power of attorney. A clearly defined legal document such as this will limit any liability that the health-care provider may incur, in caring for the patient. If the patient chooses someone outside of his or her family, the family may become upset and attempt to sue the physician, should the physician comply with the patient's wishes. However, with a signed power of attorney, the health-care provider's liability is greatly reduced, if not completely eliminated.

It is advisable for the health-care worker to determine if the patient has signed a power of attorney, or not. If one has been enacted, or the patient decides to enact one, a copy should be obtained for medical records. It is also recommended that a copy be placed in the patient's chart to provide guidance for others who work with the patient. This document makes it easier to contact the attorney-in-fact, in the event of an emergency, as their telephone numbers are listed on it.

Medical powers of attorney are a simple way to help patients maintain control over their lives following an AIDS diagnosis. Many patients perceive that by signing such a document, they are giving up control of their lives. In discussing the enactment of a power of attorney with the patient, the health-care provider can advise the patient that, by doing so, it is the *patient* who designates who will control his treatments. It should be noted, however, that the health-care provider should refer any specific questions to a legal advisor. Thus, the patient can choose someone who will carry out his wishes, rather than allowing the law to decide. It can be psychologically important to patients to realize that they still have control over their treatment, even if they themselves cannot make the decisions involved. By actively involving patients in their own care, attorneys-in-fact are provided with a guide when they must act on a patient's behalf.

In the case of an AIDS diagnosis, powers of attorney can be especially helpful when the patient has enacted a *living will*. This is a document that states that the patient does not want extraordinary medical procedures to prolong his life. Although a patient may sign such a document, health-care providers cannot simply point to the living will and disconnect machines. They *must* have the compliance of the decisionmaker. The attorney-in-fact should be familiar with the patient's wishes and, with the health-care professional's guidance regarding the patient's condition, will be able to make an informed decision on the patient's behalf.

A *legal power of attorney* allows the attorney-in-fact to conduct all legal business on behalf of a patient. Some examples are signing checks, paying bills and helping with government checks and insurance claims. Essentially, it allows the attorney-in-fact do everything that the patient can do, with his signature. This document is recommended to allow the attorney-in-fact to assist the patient to carry on with his life; especially if the patient is hospitalized and unable to do it himself.

In all cases, the attorney-in-fact should be chosen very carefully. PWAs should discuss, in depth, what their wishes and desires are, with both their attorney-in-fact and their physician. In many instances, neither the health-care provider, nor the attorney-in-fact are told what the patient really wants, and must struggle with many of the decisions to be made.

A power of attorney works in conjunction with a *last will*. A power of attorney always ends at the patient's death. However, the patient's last will becomes valid, once it is filed with a probate court, following his death. These two documents act in concert to provide someone with the authority to act on the PWAs behalf.

Last Wills

It is highly recommended that PWAs have a last will. A will allows PWAs to control where their property goes after they die. If the PWA has a lover and/or friends to whom he would like to bequeath property, a will is the only way to ensure that those persons will receive that property.

Should an individual die without a will, it is called *intestacy*. This means that, by law, the PWA's next of kin will receive his property, whether or not this is what the deceased had desired. The law looks to see if the patient was married at the time of death. If so, the spouse generally inherits all of the property. In some jurisdictions, even if a will was enacted, a spouse may have an automatic right to a share of the estate. If the patient was not married, the law looks to, in descending order, whether there are children; if not, the patient's parents would inherit. If the parents are not living, the law then looks to siblings, and so on. While some patients may want their families to get certain possessions, they may also want a partner and/or friends to receive part of their estates, as well. Because partners and friends have no legal rights, PWAs must enact wills to give them those rights. The act of making a will can be empowering to PWAs because it enables them to retain a measure of control, and it should not be thought of as morbid, or "giving up" on life.

It is extremely important for PWAs to enact their wills as early as possible. Should a patient sign a will while he is very ill, it is more likely that it may be *contested*, or challenged in court. To contest a will, someone must prove that another individual forced the patient to sign it, to that individual's benefit, or to prove that the patient was not mentally competent to enact the will. If the party that contests the will can prove one or both of these allegations, the will could be overturned, and the patient's wishes not followed. Therefore, the medical professional may want to document the patient's mental status in the patient's medical record—especially if the professional is aware that the patient is in the process of signing a will.

Living Wills

A *living will* is a declaration by patients, signed, dated, and witnessed, that essentially states that they do not want their lives prolonged artificially if they are in a hopeless, terminal condition. It is important to note that anyone involved in the patient's medical care cannot be a witness to the signature. Not all states have enacted statutes that allow living wills, but many have court decisions that address the issue, and each state has different requirements. Health-care providers should familiarize themselves with their jurisdictions' laws regarding living wills. Most laws impose certain obligations on health-care providers to certify that extraordinary measures are all that will keep the patient alive, and that the condition will be terminal within a short period of time.

A living will does not mean that a doctor can simply stop all treatments for a patient. The medical professional must also receive permission from the decisionmaker or the holder of the medical power of attorney, despite the fact that the patient has signed the document. Without such permission, the doctor must use all measures at his or her disposal to keep the patient alive. The health-care provider should have a copy of this document and discuss, with the patient, the patient's intentions and desires.

Recently, several states have acted to clarify their laws because the laws were too confusing. Under most laws, a medical professional must provide sustenance (food) and pain medication, if needed. Many statutes specifically bar invasive procedures, but require sustenance and pain control. If a patient is unconscious, it may be impossible to provide them with what is required by law without using an invasive procedure. Ideally, this would be drafted into the living will, but often it is not. The health-care provider is then caught in a legal dilemma. It is advisable to discuss, with patients, whether they want to allow limited invasive procedures, such as intravenous feeding and pain relief. The patient's response should then be documented in the chart.

Employment Discrimination

Forty-seven of the fifty states, plus the District of Columbia, have handicap discrimination laws, that prohibit discrimination based on a handicap in an employment setting. The *Federal Rehabilitation Act of 1973*[1] and the *Americans With Disabilities Act of 1990*[2] protect persons at the federal level. In the majority of state jurisdictions, as well as at the federal level, AIDS and HIV infection have been determined to be handicapping or perceived handicapping conditions. Therefore, PWAs, and in many cases HIV-positive persons and persons perceived to have HIV or AIDS, are protected in the workplace once they have a job. The federal laws, and most state laws, provide protection for those believed to be handicapped. If an employer believes that a person has AIDS and fires him, that person is protected. Even though the person may not actually have had AIDS, or have been be HIV-positive, the employer perceived that the person was infected and discriminated against him on the basis of those perceptions. In this manner, persons who are symptomatic for AIDS (formerly called AIDS Related Complex or ARC) and asymptomatic HIV seropositive individuals are also protected.

PWAs must be able to perform their jobs to have protection under the law. The law states that these persons must be "otherwise qualified" to do their jobs.[3] Therefore, if PWAs can do their jobs, despite having AIDS, protection is offered. The difficulty arises when they cannot do their jobs, or cannot be at work often enough to perform their jobs adequately. However, employers must offer *reasonable accommodation*[4] to handicapped employees. This means that employers must take action to help the employees do their jobs. This may include reducing work hours, adjusting work schedules and other measures. However, these employees must be paid the same, and lose no seniority or other rights to which they are entitled. It must, however, be economically feasible for the employer to do this. Therefore, the employer can justify firing the employee by proving that any reasonable accommodation would be too costly.

An employer cannot require any employee, or prospective employee, to take an HIV antibody test for the purpose of employment, if the purpose is to discriminate. Under very few circumstances can the employer test for employment purposes. Similarly, most employers have no legal right to an individual's confidential medical information, unless the individual is actively or casually infectious, as in the case of tuberculosis. However, if a PWA decides to tell the employer about his condition, he places the employer on notice that he is, in fact, handicapped, and the employer must accommodate the handicapping condition.

In health-care settings, legal coverage is somewhat different. Depending on the medical professional's job, the employer may be able to require HIV antibody tests. PWAs or seropositive individuals may not be able to hold certain positions, such as surgeon or operating room nurse. This also varies by jurisdiction. However, the federal Occupational Safety Health Administration (OSHA) standards[5] apply to all health-care settings. Most positions in the medical setting are similar to other employment situations, and the law will protect the health-care worker.

Insurance Issues

Insurance is one of the most complicated areas of the AIDS legal field. PWAs may have health, life and disability insurance through their place of work, or they may have an individual insurance policy. Most insurance policies, particularly health insurance policies, are issued through an individual's employer. Complications in regard to insurance may arise when an individual chooses, for whatever reason, to change jobs.

Health insurance companies may attempt to deny or limit coverage because of a *preexisting condition*. A preexisting condition means that a person was being treated for a medical condition, in a certain time period, before their policy became effective. In regard to AIDS, generally, if an individual only tests HIV-positive, and has received no treatments, it should not be considered a preexisting condition. In reality, however, many insurance companies are regarding a positive test result as a preexisting condition; even if no treatment has been rendered. Health-care providers must determine how they will accommodate such medical information in their records. If the professional has advised some treatment, or, as has been the case, has only discussed AIDS with a patient, an insurer may argue that this is, indeed, treatment, and therefore preexisting. If no treatment has been rendered, most insurers, if challenged, will cover the individual, as most states define preexisting condition to mean receiving treatment for a condition.

If a patient has a positive test result, and has received treatment for some symptoms of AIDS or ARC, they are considered to have a preexisting condition and, therefore, will not be covered. In a group policy, there is a specific preexisting period, generally 10 to 12 months, when the individual will not be covered by the health plan. However, in most states, the patient will be covered once the preexisting condition period has passed; including treatment for full-spectrum AIDS. Some states allow insurers to exclude AIDS, totally or partially; other states specifically bar the exclusion of AIDS, just as they would any other disease.

Health-care providers should be aware that their medical records are usually available to insurance companies when the patient applies for insurance because the applicant must sign release forms. If the patient has been voluntarily been tested, with a positive result, such information could harm the patient. This is an ethical, if not a legal problem, for medical personnel, as they want all pertinent medical information in their records. Due to the potential harm to patients, many doctors, and other health-care providers, have opted not to include a positive result in their records. Some insurance companies have threatened to sue for fraud, but no suits on this issue have, as yet, been filed.

If a patient is tested by a physician, is positive, and that information is entered into the medical records that are released to an insurer, or if an insurer tests the individual directly, with a positive result, several things may occur. First, the patient will be denied insurance, usually in writing. Because the insurer will release medical findings only to a physician, many people may not even know *why* they were rejected. Therefore, these individuals must write to the company and request a copy of the findings be sent to their personal physician. Second, few companies provide counseling of any kind in regard to test results. It is left to physicians to provide this type of counseling.

Finally, many insurers, particularly life insurance companies, belong to a network known as the Medical Information Bureau (MIB), located in Boston, Massachusetts. The MIB was established by the insurance companies to collect medical information about potential applicants; much as a credit bureau collects financial information. The MIB is governed by the same laws as credit bureaus. People have the right to know what is in their files and, either correct inaccurate information, or place their own personal statement in the file. Most insurance companies, if made aware of a positive HIV antibody test, will report that information to the MIB. Once this appears in an MIB file, that person's chances of obtaining insurance, anywhere in the country, are greatly diminished, if not impossible.

General Information on Insurance

Insurance companies are regulated from state to state and, therefore, an individual's rights will also vary. However, there are some federally mandated rights if a patient has group health coverage. In 1986, a federal law called *Consolidated Omnibus Budget Reconciliation Act* (COBRA)[6] took effect. This law allows people to continue their health insurance for 18 months after leaving their job unless they leave the job due to disability. The continuation period is then extended to 29 months. If an employer has 20 or more employees and is not associated with the federal government, that employer must provide the individual with the option of continuing his health insurance coverage, at his own expense, when he leaves the company. An employee can be denied this option only for gross misconduct.

Continuation means that the employee is eligible for all of the same health benefits, such as prescriptions, dental or eye care, as everyone who still works for the company. If there is an "open season" at work, and the employees can choose a new insurance company, the person on COBRA who has continued his or her insurance also can choose because the right to coverage is retained under COBRA. Finally, COBRA sets a limit on the amount of the premium. The law states that the person who wishes to continue his insurance can be charged only 102 percent of the current premium during the first 18 months, regardless of who is paying the premium while the individual is employed. If a person leaves on disability and wishes to extend coverage for the full 29 months, the cost rises to a maximum of 150 percent of the premium for the additional 11 months. It should be noted that at the end of 29 months of disability, a person becomes eligible for *Medicare*.

Many states are beginning programs which allow a person to retain his COBRA coverage but have the premium paid by Medicaid. In order to take this option, the person must be Medicaid eligible. If the person is eligible, he can apply to have his premium paid by Medicaid if the state where he lives has such a program.

COBRA affects only health insurance. Depending on the policy, people may not be able to continue on disability or life insurance benefits if they leave their job and are not disabled. If they are disabled, they will be able to utilize their disability benefits and will retain them as long as they remain disabled. Additionally, they will not have to pay the premium. Most life insurance policies allow patients to apply for a "disability waiver," which means that they will not have to pay the premium for their life insurance if they can prove that they are disabled. The patients' employer or life insurance company will be able to tell these individuals if they have this benefit, or not.

COBRA is extremely important for person with HIV disease, regardless of the stage of the disease, if they want to either leave their jobs on disability, or change jobs. If they become ill and decide to leave on disability, COBRA provides them with important health insurance coverage that they might not otherwise have including prescription coverage. Although they must pay the premiums for the coverage, it is well worth the expense because it is often difficult to qualify for Medicaid. However, if one does qualify for Medicaid, that person may be eligible for Medicaid to pay his insurance premiums. If the patient decides to change jobs and is HIV positive and/or symptomatic, the patient has a preexisting condition for the new employer's health-care plan. A new provision in COBRA gives the HIV-infected person who leaves one job and takes another the option to continue his health policy from the first job as long as he pays the appropriate premium. This is important because some policies limit or exclude coverage of preexisting conditions while others have a waiting period for preexisting conditions before coverage is effective.

COBRA allows people to continue their coverage for either 18 months or 29 months. At the end of that time, they will usually have the option to convert the group insurance policy to an individual policy at their own expense. Generally, the premium will be much higher, and almost all coverage, except medical coverage, will end. Unless a person has low income, in most cases, it is best to keep the converted insurance policy because Medicaid eligibility is difficult.

Health-care providers can greatly assist PWAs if an insurer refuses to cover a given treatment. Often an insurer will reconsider adverse decisions if patients, with their doctor's help, can properly present new or different information regarding the situation to the company.

Government Benefits

Government benefits are especially important to persons with AIDS. These benefits are provided by either a federal, state or local government, and are usually administered by the state. Some people are entitled to these benefits because they have worked and paid into the system through taxes; most are determined by disability and income. While some people may have health and life insurance through their employer, many people do not have disability insurance. If a patient becomes so sick that he is unable to continue working, benefits such as Social Security may be his only source of income. If the patient does not have health insurance, or loses it because he cannot afford to pay premiums, Medicaid may cover medical expenses.

Most PWAs experience a drastic decline in their income after diagnosis. Eventually, more than 60 percent become eligible for most government benefits because they fall below federal poverty levels. There are also other programs that may help a patient survive, such as Food Stamps, general public assistance and drug subsidy programs, even if he is on a limited income.

Social Security

There are two separate Social Security programs for disabled persons who are unable to work. Supplemental Social Income (SSI) is similar to a welfare program for disabled persons with little or no income or resources. Social Security Disability Income (SSDI) is more like an insurance program that depends on how long a person has worked, his age and income. To qualify for either of these programs, one must be considered "disabled." An explanation of the term "disabled," for Social Security purposes, is necessary. SSDI has a five-month waiting period after a person applies for benefits.

Patients with a full-blown AIDS diagnosis are considered presumptively disabled for SSI and SSDI. However, if the diagnosis is AIDS Related Complex (ARC), Social Security will consider, on a case-by-case basis, whether or not a person is able to work. In these cases, it is extremely important for the health-care provider to document fully both the disabling conditions and how these conditions prevent the patient from working. This is the criteria Social Security uses to determine whether a person is disabled. If a patient has ARC, it is vital that he seeks assistance in filling out the forms to help him meet the definition of disabled. The medical professional has an opportunity to help the patient as much as possible in this situation.

Finally, the patient must be "not working." By this stricture, Social Security requires income of less than $300 per month. The patient cannot be at the job every day, as if he was still employed full time.

SSI. To qualify for SSI, patients must be disabled and have very little in the way of income. If they meet the above definition of disabled, then they must have a very small income (generally less than $400 per month, though this figure changes periodically). Finally, their resources must be less than $2000 (this figure is also subject to change). There are certain exemptions to this, such as the total value of the patient's home, personal clothing and furniture, a car, up to a certain amount (or the whole value of the car if it is used to transport the patient to where he receives medical treatment), and a sum for funeral expenses (plus any burial plots or prepaid funeral contracts). A patient can receive SSI generally only during the five-month waiting period for SSDI. Also, if a patient lives in one of many jurisdictions, he will automatically get Medicaid coverage, if he qualifies for SSI.

SSDI. If a person has AIDS, it will be six months from the time he applies before he receives his first check. SSDI is received regardless of income from sources other than work, because the patient has paid into the system, as with any other insurance program. The amount received depends on how long a person has worked and has paid into the system, that person's age, and his income while he was working. Generally, benefits range from $400 to $900 per month, but the amount received depends on the above factors.

If the patient has been disabled for a period of 24 months, he will become eligible for Medicare (as opposed to Medicaid). A description of these two insurance programs follows.

Medicaid/Medicare

These two programs are designed to help pay medical bills when a person is disabled, has a low income, and/or does not have health insurance. There are significant differences between the two programs.

Medicaid is a joint federal—state health insurance program that is designed to provide basic medical services to eligible disabled, blind, aged and poor persons.

The eligibility criteria for Medicaid differ from state to state. Some of the medical services covered by Medicaid also differ. There are some services which are "mandatory," that is, they must be provided in every state. These services include

- Inpatient hospital care
- Outpatient care
- Physician services
- Laboratory and x-ray services
- Skilled nursing services if the patient is over 21 years old
- Home health care if the patient is eligible for skilled nursing services

A patient must meet certain income and resource guidelines to qualify for Medicaid. These guidelines also vary from state to state. Even if one has more income and resources than the guidelines allow, one can still apply and become eligible under a program called "spend down." Spend down is a criterion for eligibility that means that medical bills are large enough to bring a person's income and resources down to the levels specified within the guidelines. The patient does not have to pay the medical bills; he just has to incur the bills by receiving the medical services. These bills must then be submitted to Medicaid, and the patient must apply to qualify through spend down. There are exemptions to the resource list such as a home and car (if either is used for medical purposes). Also, if a PWA is saving money to help pay for treatment, or to pay for a drug or equipment such as a wheelchair, a certain portion can be exempted for this purpose.

Medicare is a federal health program that provides coverage for hospitalization, doctor's care and limited nursing home and home health services, for both the elderly and disabled persons. People are eligible for Medicare coverage if they are disabled, even if they are not elderly. A patient becomes eligible after receiving SSDI benefits for two years. In effect, this means a PWA must wait 29 months after diagnosis, due to the five-month waiting period for SSDI. Unfortunately, not many persons with AIDS have been able to take advantage of this program because of the long waiting period. Although this situation is changing due to medical advances in treating AIDS and its complications, the time period is still a great deal of time to wait for benefits. Furthermore, Medicare has a premium that must be paid. Generally, the premium is deducted from the SSDI check. However, if the PWA is receiving Medicaid, the Medicaid program may pay the Medicare premium for him until Medicaid no longer covers him.

AIDS Drug Subsidy Programs

The only approved anti-AIDS drug presently on the market is AZT. The typical cost of this drug is about $700 per month. However, there are also many other drugs used to treat AIDS-related illnesses, and new anti-AIDS drugs are close to being approved for distribution. Most PWAs are unable to afford these amounts, so a program was established to help them pay for drugs. This federally funded, state-administered program is designed to help persons with HIV infection pay for AZT and other drugs if they have no health insurance or their health insurance does not cover prescriptions. The scope of this coverage varies from state to state. This program was initially funded for one year, but so far it has been renewed by the government because it has helped many people receive the necessary drugs.

Food Stamps

This is a federal assistance program that provides coupons that are redeemable for food. The program is administered by the individual states. To be eligible, a PWA must meet both an asset test and an income test. If one is disabled, there is a specific income test which will apply to help them become eligible for food stamps. As with most other programs, certain items, such as a home, are exempt from the asset test.

General Public Assistance/Welfare

If a patient has ARC, and is found to be medically ineligible for SSI benefits, yet is too ill to work, he can apply for public assistance while an appeal of the SSI denial is pending. The eligibility guidelines and amount paid per month will vary from state to state. Generally, the monthly benefit is so meager that is only useful when the individual has absolutely no other resources.

Rental Assistance Programs

Many cities offer programs designed to help PWAs remain in their own homes, through rental subsidies. The PWA must apply to the city and meet income and asset guidelines to be eligible. In some cases, the landlord must agree to participate in the program. Otherwise it cannot be implemented. Most landlords, however, will agree to participate because, by doing so, they are then guaranteed that the rent, or at least a portion of it, will be paid by the city. If a PWA knows that his income is dropping, he should apply for this benefit quickly, before getting too far behind in rent payments. Once landlords have agreed to participate, it is difficult for them to evict the tenant, for the city will usually hold them to the arrangement.

Some cities offer a related program which helps pay the rent if the PWA receives an eviction notice. However, the PWA must be able to show an ability to pay the rent in the future. As a rule, the agency will take a copy of his Social Security check or, if the patient is in the waiting period, a copy of the letter granting benefits. The agency will then pay the back rent and, thus, prevent eviction.

It should be noted here, that, both the Federal Rehabilitation Act and the

Federal Housing Act of 1989, prohibit discrimination based on HIV infection. Therefore, the PWA cannot be evicted simply because of his medical condition.

The Issue of Consent

A patient has legal rights concerning his treatment that have been recognized for generations. One of these is the right to be fully informed of, and consent to, any treatment or tests which a health-care provider plans to use. This is known as the *doctrine of informed consent*. Health-care providers must understand this legal doctrine in order to provide such information to their patients, and fully informed decisions can ultimately be made by the patients or their agents.

The concept of the "health-care provider" is an ever-expanding concept. Traditionally, a health-care provider has been a physician, a dentist or a nurse. However, this concept has grown to include home health-care workers, occupational and physical therapists, social workers, or any number of others involved with the care of the patient, including family members (for the purpose of this chapter, "family" will include any person who is most significant to the patient). Health-care, itself, is a changing field, with the focus shifting from the treatment of disease, in the past, to a new trend of disease prevention.

The nature of the health-care provider—patient relationship is one of personal service by the health-care provider, unless some other arrangement has been expressly agreed upon. This relationship imposes a legal requirement on the provider to conform to the medical standards of knowledge, training, experience, skill, diligence and due care, for the patient's well-being. It also imposes a duty of confidentiality, both by court decisions and statutes. Finally, the health-care provider acts as a fiduciary to whom the patient entrusts his care.

Patients often expect their doctor, or other health-care personnel, to have all the answers. Frequently, the provider can offer nothing more than a qualified medical opinion. Thus, an inherent conflict arises between patient expectations, and the knowledge and treatment that a professional can actually deliver. The two will often coincide. However, problems may arise when they do not.

The number of malpractice suits against doctors, and others, is rapidly increasing. A patient who sues has a greater chance of success if the health-care provider failed fully to inform the patient of all of the options and treatments available, as well as the advantages and disadvantages of each option.

The Duty to Inform the Patient

Consent to Treatment

Since the turn of the century, it has been a general rule that a physician must provide patients with enough information for them to make sound judgments concerning their own medical treatment; this is the patient's right to self determination of his own health. Failure to inform a patient fully could result in misunderstandings on the part of the patient, and subsequent lawsuits. Initially, legal rulings against physicians, in this area, were based on assault and battery principles. The modern trend, however, has been to treat such acts as negligence on the part of the physician, rather than as assault and battery. There is also a tendency to include other professionals, such as nurses and anesthesiologists, in the negligence lawsuit.

Many states now have codified rulings that specify what information physicians must give their patients. Some federal regulations require that certain information be given to a patient before any procedures can be performed if the treatment is federally funded. Truly informed consent by the patient, acting on the sound advice of his health-care providers, can help a great deal in reducing the possibility of conflict by fully enabling the patient to make his decision, and to understand what the inherent risks are. It will further the provider-patient relationship, if consent to additional treatment is based on trust, and not suspicion.

Implied Consent

It is important to make the distinction between implied consent and informed consent. *Implied consent* allows a health-care provider to administer a treatment to a patient under certain circumstances. For example, if a patient is brought, unconscious, into an emergency room, and requires immediate treatment, consent to that treatment is implied by law. The patient's ability to give consent is absent in such circumstances. A court would assume that the patient would expressly authorize treatment to protect his life if he could. Implied consent in a medical emergency dictates that treatment must be provided on the basis of what is in the patient's best medical interest, and neither the patient, nor someone acting on his behalf, is able to give express consent. An emergency exists when there is an immediate threat to the life, person or health of the patient, and he may be jeopardized if treatment is delayed.

Implied consent also applies when patients present themselves for treatment and do not object to the treatment given. Many hospitals have patients sign general consent forms before rendering treatment. By signing the consent form, the hospital can argue, the patient consents to any tests or treatments that are given. This issue has become controversial with regard to HIV antibody testing. Patients may be tested without realizing it. Due to the adverse consequences associated with AIDS, it is strongly recommended that both hospitals and doctors' offices receive express consent, by signed form, before performing HIV antibody tests.

Implied consent is often statutory or regulatory in nature. For example, many states authorize breath alcohol, or even blood alcohol tests to determine the alcohol content in a driver's blood. The United States military and State Department test all applicants, active duty personnel and foreign service personnel for HIV. Those who apply for employment or membership in these institutions imply their consent to be tested, as do those who remain in their positions, knowing they will be tested.

Informed Consent

The doctrine of informed consent arose from the basis of a patient's right of self-determination in medical treatment. The majority of jurisdictions now base informed consent on the law of negligence rather than assault and battery. Even though most courts now follow the negligence theory of liability, if a health-care provider performs a procedure completely different from the one to which the patient consented, does not disclose a negative side effect which almost always occurs in non-emergency treatment, or does not disclose the experimental nature of a performed procedure, they may be liable under the battery theory.

A physician who fails to fully inform a patient of all treatments available, the risks and benefits of each treatment, and other relevant factors regarding the patient's health care is negligent in his duties as a health-care provider. The information provided must meet the applicable standard of disclosure. Generally the standard of disclosure consists of giving the patient enough information for the patient to make a reasoned, informed decision about the proposed treatment. The patient must also give authorization for the treatment.

Health-care providers must give their patients enough information for them to make an informed choice. However, it is often difficult to determine exactly how much information is necessary. The majority of jurisdictions in the United States use the professional standard; that is, to base decisions on what other health-care professionals would do in a similar situation. A growing minority, on the other hand, use the material risk standard.

The professional standard theory uses the customary disclosure practices of other physicians. The health-care provider must disclose what the reasonable physician would disclose, under the same or similar circumstances. Some courts have held that the prevailing standard to be used is the *standard of the community*[7] in which the professional is practicing. Others have used the *prevailing medical practice* theory.[8] Under the professional standard theory, a plaintiff must prove that the provider failed to meet the standard of disclosure. Often the only way to prove this is through expert testimony, which is typically hard to obtain.

Due to the difficulty in finding expert testimony, a growing number of courts have turned to the *material risk standard*. This theory is based on the premise that the patient's right to do with his body what he chooses should not be delegated by a local medical group. Courts have held that all material information must be given to the patient by the health-care provider, explaining the severity of the risk associated with the treatment, and the chance of complications occurring. The more severe the risk, the more material the reasonable person would perceive it to be. While the courts recognize that it may be unrealistic to disclose every possible risk, the provider must disclose the nature and the purpose of the treatment, the risks and benefits, as well as any alternatives.

A risk is material if it is likely to affect the patient's decision. The plaintiff does not need expert medical testimony to prove his case in states which have adopted the material risk standard. The court will allow a jury to decide what information was "material" to the reasonable patient. A minority of courts reject the reasonable standard, saying that it limits true self-determination of treatment by the patient. These courts use a subjective standard, that is, what a particular patient would consider material. Some expert testimony regarding the nature of the treatment, and the risks involved, may still be necessary in order to demonstrate the relationship between the provider's failure to disclose, and the patient's injury.

As a general rule, health-care providers should discuss all treatment, or proposed treatment, with their patients. This should include information regarding the risks and benefits of treatment, as well as possible alternatives. There are currently so many experimental treatments for AIDS that health-care providers must be particularly careful when attempting a new treatment with a given patient. Often the patient may request a certain treatment. If this is the case, the physician is obligated to learn as much as possible about the treatment, in order to direct the patient best to try the treatment or not.

Refusal to Treat

By its very nature, AIDS is a frightening disease. People are generally afraid of the unknown and, in medical circumstances, they turn to the health-care provider for guidance. Unfortunately, some health professionals have been unwilling to learn about AIDS and have reacted by refusing to treat PWAs.

Case Study

In July 1987, a man named Rod Miller cut his foot on a beach in Delaware. The cut appeared to be severe and he was taken to a hospital in Lewes, Delaware. The doctor on duty asked Mr. Miller if he had ever taken an HIV antibody test, to which Mr. Miller responded no. The doctor refused to treat him because he suspected that Mr. Miller was gay. He stated to a newspaper reporter that he was suspicious because of the "demeanor" of Mr. Miller and his friends. He continued that one of the friends was wearing a shirt that said, "Gentlemen Prefer Blondes"; the wearer happened to be a blonde. Mr. Miller was flown, by helicopter, to a hospital in Washington, DC, where he was treated. He now suffers permanent damage to his foot.

A complaint was filed with the Health and Human Services (HHS) Office of Civil Rights, Region 3, after an investigator in that office read a newspaper account of the incident and contacted Mr. Miller. The case was closed by HHS on September 9, 1989, with a confidential statement. However, HHS has publicly stated that it will not tolerate discrimination of this kind.

In many states, health-care providers and hospitals are considered "public accommodations," and are covered by the handicap discrimination statutes. A public accommodation is one that provides services to the general public. Because federal and most state laws prohibit discrimination based on HIV status, a health-care provider must have a valid reason to refuse treatment, such as a lack of knowledge or expertise with a particular symptom that a patient may exhibit. However, this cannot be used as a reason not to treat the patient at all. If the provider does not feel competent to administer treatment, he must still make a referral for the patient.

The American Medical Association (AMA) has stated that it is unethical for a medical doctor to refuse treatment of a PWA. This statement was prompted partly by the Miller case, as well as numerous other similar cases that have been reported to the AMA. The health-care provider who refuses treatment may face ethical, as well as legal, action.

Liability Issues

Health-care providers may face liability issues when treating PWAs. For example, in a California case involving a mental health counselor, it was ruled that the provider was liable to the family of one of his patient's friend, for wrongful death. The counselor failed to notify the friend that the patient had threatened to murder her; in fact, the patient carried out the threat.[9] Although the provider had taken action by alerting the local police, the court ruled that he should have done more by warning the potential victim directly. In an AIDS setting, a PWA may inform his doctor that he is continuing to have unprotected sex with unsuspecting partners. The California case, which has been followed around the country, implies that the doctor has a potential obligation to warn those who might be affected by a patient's behavior. To date, there have been no civil cases that directly address this issue. However, many factors must be considered: Can a partner be identified by the doctor? Given the long incubation period of AIDS, can a doctor be held liable for something that might happen 15 years in the future? Should the doctor give the patient's name to public health authorities? Finally, is this enough to shield the doctor from liability?

Because no cases have, as yet, been decided, health-care providers are in a state of turmoil and confusion regarding this issue. Some general guidelines may help. The health-care provider should first ascertain what knowledge the patient has about AIDS. If a PWA does not realize that he is potentially harming others, information about the disease may help the patient alter his behavior. If the patient is knowledgeable about AIDS and still does not want to change, the doctor should warn him that, as a physician, he has some obligation to protect the public health, and attempt to convince that patient to alter his behavior.

The AMA has stated that the public health danger of being infected (with HIV) is great enough to justify breaking a patient's confidentiality. If a patient refuses to change his behavior, the doctor may have an obligation to inform public health authorities. In addition, if one or more partners can be identified, the doctor may have an obligation to warn them, as well. The doctor must take reasonable steps to ensure the public safety; this responsibility, then, limits his liability. However, it is advisable that health-care personnel check their local laws, as some may prohibit disclosure, except by court order, while others may restrict breaking a patient's confidentiality in other ways. It is vital for health-care personnel to know this information in case they are ever presented with a similar situation.

Conclusion

AIDS is challenging health-care providers in ways never before imagined. On one hand, there is an active, well-educated patient group demanding better treatment and access to drugs faster than medicine can accommodate. On the other hand, minorities, who unfortunately have traditionally lacked access to adequate health-care, and are increasingly becoming infected with HIV, are now straining the system, both medically and financially. No other single disease has caused quite the social stir that AIDS has, and health-care professionals are often caught in the middle. By staying well informed about new treatments, and by keeping abreast of the rapidly changing medical, legal and social implications of the disease, modern medical professionals will be able to continue to provide the quality medical care to which we have become accustomed.

References

1. Federal Rehabilitation Act of 1973, 29 U.S.C. Sec 504, as amended, 29 U.S.C. Sec 794.

2. Pub. L. 101-336, 104 Stat. 327 (1990). To be codified at 42 U.S.C. Sec. 12101. A.D.A. differs from the Federal Rehabilitation Act in that a program or organization does not need to receive federal money to be covered. After July 26, 1994, the A.D.A. will cover all employers who have 15 or more employees. From July 26, 1992, all employers with more than 25 employees will be covered. Otherwise the coverage between the two federal Acts is similar in the discrimination protections offered.

3. 29 U.S.C. Sec 504, Pub. L. 93-112, Title V, Sec 504, 87 Stat. 394 (1973) [applicable version, including 1986 amendments, at 29 U.S.C. 794 (West Supp. 1990)]. Sec 504 states, "No otherwise qualified handicapped individual in the United States as defined in Section 7(6), shall, solely by reason of his handicap, be excluded from the participation in, be denied benefits of, or be subjected to discrimination under any program or activity receiving Federal financial assistance."

4. 29 U.S.C.A. Sec 794 states, "Otherwise qualified handicapped individual must be provided with meaningful access to the benefit which the governmental grantee offers; the benefit itself cannot be defined in a way that effectively denies otherwise qualified handicapped individuals the meaningful access to which they are entitled; to ensure meaningful access, **reasonable accommodations** in the grantee's program or benefit may have to be made." (Emphasis added.) See also, *Alexander v. Choate*, 469 U.S. 287, 105 S.Ct. 712 (1985).

5. 29 U.S.C.A. Sec. 651.

6. Consolidated Omnibus Budget Reconciliation Act of 1985, 29 U.S.C.A. Sec. 1162 (1986).

7. *Roberts v. Young*, 119 N.W.2d 627, 369 Mich. 133 (1963).

8. *Dietze v. King*, 184 F. Supp. 944 (1960).

9. *Tarasoff v. Regents of the University of California*, 131 Cal. Rptr. 14, 551 P.2d 334 (1976).

14 AIDS Education
Stopping AIDS, Stopping Fear

William M. Marcil, MS, OTR

We have nothing to fear but fear itself.
—Franklin Delano Roosevelt
You can't fight a moral problem by ignoring it.
—Harry S. Truman

Introduction

Throughout history people have been afraid of the unknown; it seems to be part of our nature. When we encounter a person of another race or culture for the first time, we are nervous and wary. When embarking on a trip to a new place or to begin a new job, we do so with a great deal of trepidation and apprehension. When we see a disheveled, homeless man acting in a bizarre manner on the street, we cross to the other side. In these and countless other novel situations, we act as we do because we do not completely understand what is happening. We feel out of control. We feel afraid and we react to that fear in ways that are individualized, yet common to others.

Since the turn of the century, and particularly in the years following World War II, medical science has successfully eradicated or controlled many of the diseases that have plagued the human race for centuries. With the exception of polio, for which a vaccine was developed in the mid-1950s, we have had relatively few diseases to be concerned about. Certainly, a cure for cancer continues to elude us, for now. However, even many forms of that disease can now be controlled or even cured. We have become, by and large, complacent in a relatively healthy lifestyle.

The advent of AIDS has reintroduced us to the fear that a disease can produce as its by-product. We have responded to that fear with the same defense mechanisms that our ancestors used: denial, hostility, intolerence, isolationism, and ignorance (maybe it will go away). Not only must we deal with a relentless and deadly disease, but we have also been forced to address other issues that we have also denied and avoided over the years: homosexuality, IV drug use and the premature death of a relatively young population.

As in the past, and certainly in the course of our daily activities, we overcome our fears by becoming familiar with and facing them head-on. While animals can react to their fears, both real and perceived, with only instinct and limbic functions, people can overcome their fears by the higher cognitive function of learning. When we learn about anything, we become familiar with it by examining and exploring all of its possiblities. We are then able to integrate that information and make a volitional choice either to use that knowledge or disregard it in the future. Our learning and knowledge is achieved through the education process.

The Fear

In the early 1980s, earliest days of the epidemic, virtually nothing was known about AIDS—what caused it, how it was spread, or how to care for its victims. In fact, it did not even have a name. Because gay men were the primary population at risk at that time, it was referred to as GRIDS, or gay-related immune deficiency syndrome. Initially, knowledge of the disease was sparse; largely because of the small select group of people affected. Only physicians working with large numbers of gay men were concerned about this strange disease and got little, if any, assistance from colleagues and government agencies.

With the number of AIDS cases growing daily, the apprehension of the gay community began to mount in direct proportion. Individuals who had little or no familiarity with medical issues and terminology began to educate themselves about the immune system and the opportunistic diseases that ravaged their friends and lovers. Despite this knowledge, The Fear within the gay community ran rampant. There was still no known cause for the disease. Theories ranged from stimulants used to enhance sexual pleasure (poppers) to different lubricants used during anal intercourse. The lack of knowledge about the disease was disconcerting and The Fear among gays raged. Within the general population, however, the disease remained virtually unheard of.

As the incidence of this baffling disease increased at a steady rate, small, isolated groups of researchers began taking an interest in this anomaly and, in 1984, the cause, a virus (HTLV-III/LAV; now HIV), was finally isolated. This identification was the first step in effectively combatting the disease. From this knowledge, the modes of transmission could be determined. Unfortunately, there was no way to know who was, or how many were, infected. However, based on what was now known, the concept of safer sex was conceived as a method of reducing transmission.

The heterosexual majority, however, remained relatively ignorant about AIDS and, with the exception of health-care personnel, felt that they had no need for such information; it didn't concern them. For those health-care workers, however, AIDS was becoming a major concern. AIDS was seen as a contagious disease that killed people and PWAs in the hospital were treated as if they were less than human. Many were given inappropriate, substandard care by hospital personnel afraid of contracting the disease. Despite what was known about AIDS transmission, the fear of contagion persisted.

It was not until the mid-1980s, mostly due to increasing media coverage, that the general public began to take an interest in this "new" disease called AIDS, although no one seemed overly concerned. However, with the 1985 death of Rock Hudson, who, to many, was the epitome of masculinity and heterosexuality, public concern was ignited. Although Hudson's "secret" lifestyle was confirmed after his death, it was soon common knowledge that AIDS was not just a disease of homosexuals; heterosexuals could contract it, as well. The Fear, which had previously been rampant only in the gay community, took hold of the general population with lightning speed. It was no longer safe to have casual sexual encounters, to kiss, or even to touch one of questionable sexuality. Waiters with suspect sexual preference were avoided, for fear of contracting AIDS by casual contact or by eating off of contaminated utensils. Opportunists took advantage of The Fear and marketed products that allegedly prevented the transmission of AIDS. One such item was a disposable cover for telephone mouthpieces that may have been previously used by an infected individual. A seat on a crowded bus was left unoccupied because a prankster had scrawled, "The last person to sit here had AIDS." In San Francisco, a man was beaten and forced off of a bus because some other passengers thought that he had Kaposi's lesions on his face. In just a few short months, society had dramatically changed. The Fear had taken over.

Much of The Fear has abated in recent years, but not all of it. To be sure, a little fear is a good thing, for AIDS is certainly something of which we should be afraid. However, despite all of the recent knowledge about AIDS—how it is spread, how it is not spread—unnecessary fear continues to persist in a substantial segment of the general population and, surprisingly, among health-care workers, as well. The Fear has prevented health-care workers from performing their jobs adequately and therefore it must be eradicated. Just as a fire can be extinguished only by cutting off the source of its fuel supply, so can The Fear be extinguished, by cutting off its fuel supply—ignorance. The best weapon that we have both to fight The Fear and reduce the number of new HIV infections is education.

AIDS Education

AIDS education is certainly not a new concept. We are constantly exposed to ads which warn us to "be careful," to use a condom, or to "tell a friend." "AIDS does not discriminate." "AIDS is an equal opportunity destroyer." Everyone knows what AIDS is. Why, then, are more people becoming infected everyday? Why does The Fear persist? Perhaps our approach to AIDS education is an incomplete, single systems method. Perhaps our approach isn't all that it can or should be.

It has been said that much of the current AIDS information and educational material is written at the second year college level. This is all well and good if one has had the good fortune to attend at least two years of college. But what about those people who have not been to college or, for that matter, haven't even finished high school? What about our children? Teenagers are fast becoming the greatest risk group for contracting HIV.[1] There are many other groups that we must target, as well. Non-English-speaking or Spanish-speaking populations, the illiterate, the developmentally disabled, the mentally retarded, the emotionally disturbed and psychiatric populations, to cite a few examples, must be addressed. All of these groups are capable of contracting and spreading HIV, but are we reaching out to them?

We are extremely fortunate to live in a time when information can be disseminated to millions of people in a split second. A full 90 percent of the U.S. population owns at least one television set. We have access to radio, newspapers, periodicals, books and journals. In addition, we have bulletin boards, billboards, computers and telephones. These are all excellent tools for communicating information if they are used correctly and to their full potentials. Like any tool, however, they are limited in their usefulness and we must frequently employ a number of tools to complete any job effectively and efficiently. A hammer is a useful tool to use if one wishes to drive nails into two pieces of wood. However, it does not help cut those pieces to fit together in the first place. To be effective, one must use "the right tool for the right job."

Education is a tool, and so are the variety of communication modalities which we have at our disposal. If we use only a couple of the tools at our disposal, we cannot complete the task at hand. We must have a well-stocked tool box if we are to do a thorough job.

America Responds to AIDS

In 1988, the federal government sponsored a mass mailing of AIDS information to every household in the United States that supplied a great deal of basic yet important information about what AIDS is, how it is spread, how it is not spread and how to prevent further spread of the virus.[2] This was certainly a great step in educating the public about AIDS, and it was an unprecedented approach to any previous public health problem. However, this approach made number of assumptions about the people who would receive this information—that they had a permanent address, they were literate, they had no visual impairments, they could understand the information and they would take the time actually to read it. This approach is not neccesarily going to benefit those individuals who are most at risk for contracting AIDS—the homeless, IV drug users, and the like (Figure 14-1). Although this is certainly an effective and useful tool in AIDS education, it is limited in its utility.

The Use of the Media in AIDS Education

The media, television in particular, has been an extremely useful tool in AIDS education. Television has the ability to reach out to millions of people instantly. Early attempts to educate the public about AIDS via this medium were initially met with some effrontery due to the nature of the illness, the groups most at risk and the modes of transmission. The idea of advertising condoms and promoting safe sex was unheard of in the conservative broadcasting industry. Necessity and pressure, from both within and without the industry, eventually led to the airing of these unprecedented, and sometimes contoversial, messages. Some segments of the industry, however, found the concept very appealing. The so-called soap operas picked up on the issue of AIDS early on and integrated it into many of

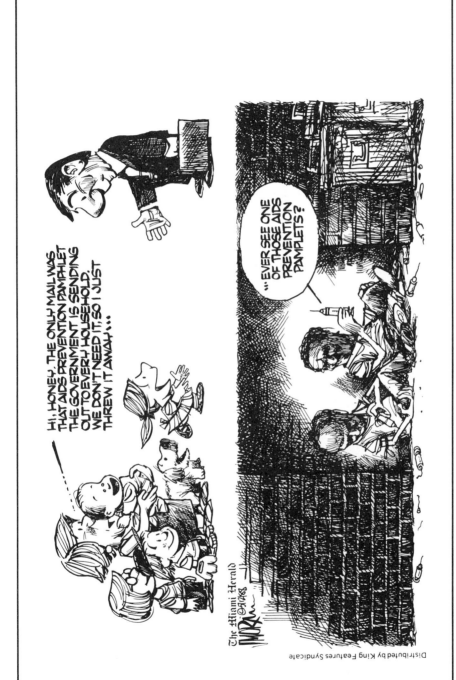

Figure 14-1. America responds to AIDS. ©1988 King Features Syndicate. Used with permission.

their story lines. Certainly, many of these shows were initially aiming at the sensationalism of the topic. However, for a genre of entertainment frequently lambasted for its liberal employment of gratuitous sex, many of these shows have, undoubtedly, succeeded in educating many viewers about AIDS in a somewhat unconventional manner.

Although it is no longer uncommon to see AIDS commercials, documentaries or dramas on television, this is not to say that all potential viewers will receive the message. Many of the AIDS commercials are not shown during the prime viewing times. Many stations reserve these for late night viewing, reaching only a limited audience. Because the ultimate decision to air any spot lies with the local station manager, many viewers may be denied access to important information based on the subjective discretion of one individual. To be sure, decisions of this nature could be made on the basis of actual or perceived public opinion. Be that as it may, we can see that even television has its limitations as a tool in AIDS education.

Returning to our toolbox analogy, if we approach a large task, building a house for example, we must have a large variety of tools at our disposal and know how to use them — if we are to complete the task at hand. In terms of AIDS education, we must also have our tools and know how to use them properly. If we do not have a particular tool to finish the job, we need to obtain it, learn how to use it and employ it in the appropriate manner. To combat the public health problem of AIDS effectively, we must utilize every possible tool at our disposal. Although the media provides us with a great deal of options, this does not appear to be the only method of AIDS education. The message is not getting across to all who are at risk for HIV infection.

AIDS Education: A Suggested Approach

As health professionals and as individuals, we have a duty and an obligation to participate in the AIDS education process in any way we can. This process involves educating ourselves, our peers and colleagues, our families and friends, our patients and their families; including those individuals who are already in some stage of HIV infection, and anyone else who has a need to know about AIDS; that is, everyone (Figure 14-2). This approach is in keeping with Fiebleman's law of the hierarchy.[3]

Self Education

Before one can educate others about AIDS, it is logical to assume that one must educate oneself about it first. This is the first phase of the AIDS education process. Because new information on this topic is made available on a daily basis, through a variety of media, it is imperative that each of us keep abreast of these changes. AIDS is not a static disease, and we cannot afford to be static in our knowledge of it if we are to be effective in the education process. By educating ourselves about AIDS, we are not only gaining more insight and knowledge, but we are also facing The Fear, and, thus, we will be able to conquer it and gradually help others to overcome it, as well.

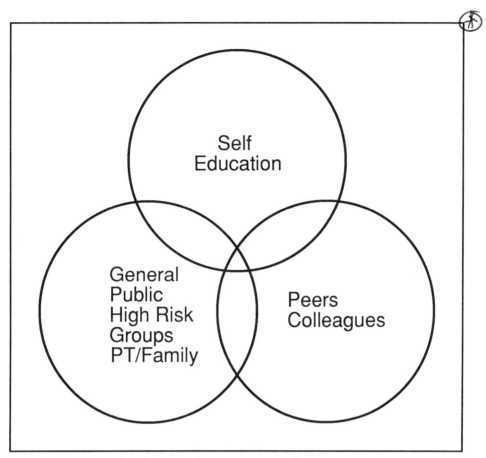

Self
Education

General
Public
High Risk
Groups
PT/Family

Peers
Colleagues

Figure 14-2. AIDS education triad. ©1990, W.M. Marcil.

Educating Colleagues and Peers

The second aspect of the education process involves sharing one's own knowledge with ones colleagues and peers. Although health professionals should be knowledgeable about AIDS, it is astounding that there are still great numbers of individuals who are uninformed, misinformed or personally biased against those individuals with the disease. There are those who believe that they will never have to encounter a person with AIDS or HIV disease and, therefore, feel that they have no need to be concerned. The fact is that we all must be prepared to deal with this population at some point in our careers. One cannot tell if a given patient is HIV positive just by looking at him. It is paramount that universal precautions be followed with *all* patients, regardless of their diagnoses.[4,5] These precautions prevent not only the transmission of HIV from an infected patient to the health-care worker, but it also prevents the transmission of other diseases, as well. Conversely, these precautions also prevent the spread of disease(s) from health-care workers to their patients. Knowledge and practice of universal precautions by all health-care workers will ultimately benefit everyone who is involved in the health-care system.

One cannot deny the fact that there have been health-care workers who have contracted HIV infection from on the job exposures;[4,6] although the true numbers may never be known, the incidence of these cases seem to be relatively low. This, however, does not seem to satisfy a number of health-care workers. Certain professionals (orthopedic surgeons, for example, who risk accidental infection from bone fragments which may pierce their gloves and skin) will always be at some degree of high risk for possible exposure, regardless of precautionary measures taken to avoid such untoward incidents. These professions must examine new ways to provide protection for their members (such as impenetrable surgical gloves) while simultaneously ensuring quality treatment for their patients. We can neither deny our patients the benefit of our knowledge and expertise because of The Fear, nor treat our patients in a cavalier manner, which may put us in jeopardy.

On the other hand, while the risk of occupational exposure exists, the truth of the matter is that everyone, health-care professionals included, stands a greater risk for contracting HIV through extracurricular activities—specifically unprotected, gratuitous sexual relationships and IV drug use. Because AIDS is frequently associated with gay men, IV drug users and minorities, individuals in other groups tend not to be as concerned about their personal recreational habits. This attitude puts these individuals at an increased risk of contracting not only HIV, but other diseases such as hepatitis, herpes, syphilis and gonorrhea, as well. Perhaps through the education process we can also reduce the risk and incidence of these diseases.

In the process of educating those who are already working in the health field, we should also include those individuals who are considering a career in the medical, nursing or allied health professions. AIDS has deterred a number of potential health-care practitioners from entering the field due to the fear of contagion. This has is most evident by decreased enrollment in nursing schools.[7] The increased incidence of AIDS is reportedly a leading cause of this decline. It is essential that the facts about AIDS reach these young people if the health industry is to remain adequately staffed into the twenty-first century.

Educating the General Public

The third and final aspect of the education process essentially targets anyone else who has a need to know about AIDS. This is an extensive group, for it should include everyone with whom one comes into contact. Everyone needs to know the facts and the myths about AIDS. Everyone needs to understand that AIDS is not a disease that "happens to others." It is not a disease of gays, or junkies or prostitutes. It is not merely a public health problem, either. It is a problem of attitudes, of moral judgment, of social issues, of politics and of economics. The disease of AIDS itself is at the subsystem level. However, as indicated by the laws of the levels, the higher levels of the hierarchy are dependent on the lower levels, and the lower is directed by the higher.[3] This is to say that the higher levels of community, society and nation are impacted by the lower level of AIDS and, conversely, the course that AIDS takes will ultimately be directed by the strategy that we as a society, nation and united humanity employ in dealing with this problem.

It is therefore crucial that each of us do our part in the fight against AIDS. With education as our best weapon in this battle, we must employ it at every opportunity. We must educate our friends and family, our neighbors, our parishoners and passing acquaintances in any way we can. "Word of mouth advertising" can often be the best method of getting a particular message across to a given special-interest group.

We must also educate those individuals who are already in some stage of HIV infection, as well as their family members and friends. Just because one is HIV-positive does not mean that he automatically knows everything there is to know about the disease. Just as a cancer patient doesn't always know what to expect from his disease, neither does the patient with AIDS, or related conditions, know what to expect. For example, if a couple who are both HIV-positive, and are now in a strictly monogomous relationship, they should be made aware that, because there are approximately 120 different subtypes of HIV, that they should continue to practice safe sex to avoid passing these different subtypes to each other, thus reducing the risk of further complications.[8] It is our duty to teach these individuals how to keep themselves healthier, how to prevent further transmission of the virus, and where to go for assistance with any problems that they might encounter.

To be sure, no one individual can know all that there is to know about AIDS and, therefore, each of us is limited in what we can do. Every tool has its limitations and we should realize what our limitations are, for fear that we may do more harm than good. For example, although outreach workers on the street are a very effective method of disseminating AIDS education in the inner city, it is unlikely that members of a given minority group are going to listen to what a white, middle-class PhD has to say to them and, therefore, information that could save their lives will fall on deaf ears. It would seem logical, then, that outreach workers of the same culture/race be utilized to accomplish the same task.

Similarly, teenagers are unlikely to take heed of what adults might have to say about AIDS; teenagers are notorious for rebellion and, at the same time, perceive themselves to be invincible to any possible harm (it should be noted that many adults feel this way as well, due to the powerful nature of the sex drive or of narcotic addiction). Unfortunately, it is these qualities that make modern teenagers one of the fastest growing risk groups for HIV disease.[1] In this instance, it makes more sense to utilize peer counselors and popular songs and music videos to get the message across to this vulnerable group. As a means of educating teenagers about AIDS, Professor Harold Cohen and his students at the State University of New York, Buffalo School of Architecture, created a mobile AIDS education unit which allows teens to utilize interactive video displays to learn the facts and myths about the disease. This van is wheelchair accessible and uses universal symbols to convey the message, rather than relying on language alone. This van is currently in use throughout New York State by the State Health Department.

The Role of Traditional Education

AIDS education in the primary and secondary school system has been heavily advocated by some groups, while it was vehemently opposed by others. This is an area that causes a great deal of consternation on both sides. If we address an issue such as AIDS to this young group, we must also address issues to which many adults do not believe that young children should be exposed— sexuality, specifically homosexuality, and IV drug use. Although it is inevitable that all children will face these topics at some point in their young lives, the question remains: At what age do we introduce these topics? How long do we protect their innocence?

On the other hand, if we do not address the topic of AIDS at some level early in the education process, we are not only doing our children a great disservice, but we are also endangering their lives. Childhood and adolescence are times of inquisitive exploration which, for good or bad, tends to include exploration of sexuality and experimentation with drugs. If they are not made aware of the possible deadly consequences of these practices, we will continue to lose our most valuable resource—and our legacy. Perhaps if we can devise an AIDS education program that is accepted by the majority, we can increase the pool of AIDS-literate school children and, it is hoped, reduce the number of future AIDS cases. This will not be an easy task, as evidenced by our inability to implement even basic sex education courses in our schools that are accepted by the majority. By addressing the issue of AIDS in a positive and effective manner, we may also be able to decrease the incidence of other sexually transmitted diseases, teenage pregnancy and drug abuse at the same time. Although this may seem to be a rather Pollyanna-ish perspective, it is worth the attempt.

The Economics of AIDS Education

There is an economic incentive to promote effective AIDS education, as well. In 1986 it was estimated that the cost of caring for the first 10,000 AIDS patients would exceed 16 billion dollars.[9] When one considers that there are now over 100,000 cases in the United States alone, and over 200,000 worldwide, one must wonder what the bottom line will be in terms of AIDS-related costs, including lost worktime. The impact of AIDS has effected the cost of everyone's medical care, our insurance rates and the taxes that we pay. As the number of AIDS cases continues to increase, so will the financial burden of caring for its victims rise in direct proportion. Although there is nothing that we can do to change the current numbers, through the education process, we can, it is hoped, decrease the number of new cases which will ease the financial strain of the disease.

Everyone Has a Role in AIDS Education

We have seen that AIDS is not just an isolated disease that affects a small, select group of people; it affects all of us in some way, shape or form. We have seen how one of the smallest, simplest forms of life, at the subsystems level, can have have an effect on the higher levels of systems and supersystems. We have also seen that, although the lower level effects the higher level, it is ultimately the higher that directs the lower. AIDS education occurs primarily at the systems level of conduct and experiences, that is, the person. It is directed by the subsystem level and, in turn, effects the supersystems of family, community, subculture, culture, society and nation. By viewing both the problem of AIDS and the educational approach to combatting it from a general systems perspective, we can gain a more objective insight into what our course(s) of action should be.

Although, currently, there is nothing that we can do to "take away" HIV disease from those who are already infected, we can attempt to take away some of their pain and suffering through scientific advancements, understanding, compassion and empathy. All of these are acquired through the education process. Education can also enable us to prevent further spread of the disease and, thus, "take it away" from future generations. Due to the nature of HIV infection and its modes of transmission, theoretically we could completely stop its proliferation through a proper educational approach. Human nature being what it is, however, makes this utopian ideal unlikely. This does not mean that we should not strive for it, just the same. Just as the incidence of AIDS has increased in a geometric progression, so can the incidence of AIDS education proliferate— one person passing it on to another person or to a group of people who, in turn, can pass it to others. Let us hope that the education process can progress further and faster than the virus itself.

Postscript

This chapter has addressed the extreme importance of AIDS education in retarding the progression of the disease. In fact, this is the basic message of the entire text—that only through education and understanding will we be able to stop the spread of this relentless disease, and also stop the fear of it, as well. AIDS education is everyone's business. We cannot bury our heads in the sand and hope that it will go away, because it won't; it will only get worse. AIDS is a fact of modern life and it will continue to be until well into the next century.

Throughout this text we have seen that AIDS is not a single systems phenomenon; it effects every level of our existence, from the simplest to the most complex. The battle against this disease is equally complex and cannot be won if we approach it by attempting to combine the multiple, yet individual parts into a more complete whole. Means to combat AIDS must first be viewed in terms of the whole to see how the various levels fit together and how they should, and must, interact as an integrated unit; rather than as separate entities speaking different languages, working to build a new "Tower of Babel."

Perhaps something beneficial will come out of this terrible tragedy called AIDS. Science frequently stumbles onto answers to many other problems in the attempt to solve a different puzzle. We have learned more about AIDS in the span of one decade than was learned about any other disease that preceded it. Perhaps in our search for a cure and/or vaccine for AIDS, we will solve other mysteries in the process: cancer, multiple sclerosis, the common cold, or, perhaps even the process of aging. Everything seems to have a purpose; why not AIDS?

We are now in the midst of a crisis, and a crisis, it is said, tends to pull people together. This is what we must do now. We must pull together to fight a common foe. We must look beyond the symptoms of the disease and the lifestyles of those who are its victims. We must pull together as a human community if we are to emerge victorious. AIDS is the foe; not its victims. AIDS is everyone's concern. AIDS is everybody's business.

References

1. Belfer, M.L., Krener, P.K., and Miller, F.B. (1988). AIDS in children and adolescents. *Journal of the American Academy of Child and Adolescent Psychiatry,* 27(2):147-151.
2. U.S. Department of Health and Human Services, U.S. Public Health Services, Centers for Disease Control (1988). *Understanding AIDS.* HHS publication no. (CDC) HHS-88-8404. Washington, DC: GPO.
3. Fiebleman, J.K. (1954). Theory of integrated levels. *British Journal for the Philosophy of Science,* (5):59-66.
4. Centers for Disease Control (1988). Update: Universal precautions for prevention of human immunodeficiency virus, hepatitis B virus, and other bloodborne pathogens in health-care settings. *Mobidity and Mortality Weekly Report,* 37(24):377.
5. Centers for Disease Control (1987). Recommendations for prevention of HIV transmision in health-care settings. *Morbidity and Mortality Weekly Report,* 36(2S):3S-4S.
6. Centers for Disease Control (1987). Update: Human immunodeficiency virus infections in health-care workers exposed to blood of infected patients. *Morbidity and Mortality Weekly Report,* 36(19):285-289.
7. National study shows sharp drop in the number of college freshmen planning nursing careers. (1987). *American Journal of Nursing,* April:530.
8. Clement, M. (1989). Patient care queries. *AIDS Clinical Care,* 1(6):54.
9. Hardy, A.M., Raugh, K., Echenberg, D., et al. (1986). The economic impact of the first 10,000 cases of acquired immune defficiency syndrome in the United States. *Journal of the American Medical Association,* 255(2):209-211.

Bibliography

Boland, M.G., Allen, T.J., Long, G.I., et al. (1988). Children with HIV infection: Collaborative responsibilities of the child welfare and medical communities. *Social Work,* November-December:504-509.

Boland, M.G., Tasker, M., Evans, P.M., et al. (1987). Helping children with AIDS: The role of the child welfare worker. *Public Welfare,* Winter:23-28.

Quackenbush, M. and Nelson, M. (1988). *The AIDS Challenge: Prevention Education for Young People.* San Francisco: San Francisco AIDS Foundation.

Quackenbush, M. and Villareal, S. (1988). *Does AIDS Hurt?: Educating Young Children About AIDS.* San Francisco: San Francisco AIDS Foundation.

Shilts, R. (1987). *And the Band Played On.* New York: St. Martin's Press.

Sroka, S.R. (1987). *Educators Guide to AIDS and other STD's.* Manor Park, NY: Health Education Consultants.

Staff (1988). *AIDS and the Education of Our Chidren.* U.S. Department of Education. Washington, DC: U.S. Government Printing Office.

Staff (1989). *Infection Precautions for People with HIV: Household Guidelines.* San Francisco: San Francisco AIDS Foundation.

Staff (1986). *Reaching Ethnic Communities in the Fight Against AIDS.* Communications Technologies and Research and Decisions Corporation.

Staff (1987). *What Parents Need to Tell Children About AIDS.* Albany, NY: New York State Department of Health.

Tasker, M. (1988). *Jimmy and the Eggs Virus.* Newark, NJ: Childrens Hospital AIDS Program.

Weiner, R. (1986). *AIDS: Impact on the Schools.* Education Research Group, Alexandria, VA: Capitol Publications.

Yarber, W.L. (1987). *AIDS Education: Curriculum and Health Policy.* Phi Delta Kappa Educational Foundation.

Suggested Readings

Alyson, S. (Ed.) (1988). *You Can Do Something About AIDS.* Boston: The Stop AIDS Project, Inc.

Cahill, K.M. (Ed.) (1983). *The AIDS Epidemic.* New York: St. Martin's Press.

Gallo, R.C. (1987). The AIDS virus. *Scientific American,* 256(1):46-56.

Hayward-Albertson, S. (1980). *Endings and Beginnings.* New York: Random House.

Kubler-Ross, E. (1987). *AIDS: The Ultimate Challenge.* New York: Macmillan.

Langone, J. (1985). AIDS. *Discover,* 6(12)(December):28-53.

Mizel, S.B. and Jaret, P. (1985). *The Human Immune System: The New Frontier in Medicine.* New York: Simon and Schuster.

Pan American Health Organization. *AIDS: Profile of an Epidemic.* Washington, DC: World Health Organization.

Piel, J. (Ed). (1988). What science knows about AIDS (special issue). *Scientific American,* 259(4):1-152.

Saunders, C. and Baines, M. (1989). *Living with Dying.* Oxford: Oxford Medical Publications.

Shilts, R. (1987). *And the Band Played On.* New York: St. Martin's Press.

Tigges, K.N. and Marcil, W.M. (1988) *Terminal and Life Threatening Illness: An Occupational Behavior Perspective.* Thorofare, NJ: Slack.

Weinberg, G.M. (1975). *An Introduction to General Systems Thinking.* New York: John Wiley & Sons.

Appendices

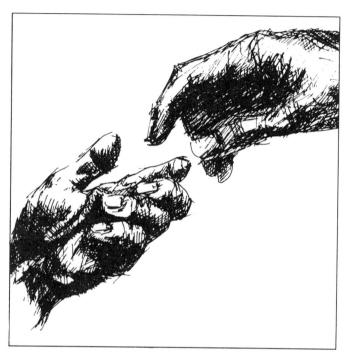

Appendix A

Revision of the CDC Surveillance Case Definition for AIDS

Council of State and Territorial Epidemiologists: AIDS
Program, Center for Infectious Diseases, CDC*

Introduction

The following revised case definition for surveillance of AIDS was developed by CDC in collaboration with public health and clinical specialists. The Council of State and Territorial Epidemiologists (CSTE) has officially recommended adoption of the revised definition for national reporting of AIDS. The objectives of the revision are 1) to track more effectively the severe disabling morbidity associated with infection with HIV (including HIV-1 and HIV-2); 2) to simplify reporting of AIDS cases; 3) to increase the sensitivity and specificity of the definition through greater diagnostic application of laboratory evidence for HIV infection; and 4) to be consistent with current diagnostic practice, which in some cases includes presumptive, that is, without confirmatory laboratory evidence, diagnosis of AIDS-indicative diseases (e.g., PCP, KS).

The definition is organized into three sections that depend on the status of laboratory evidence of HIV infection (e.g., HIV antibody). The major proposed changes apply to patients with laboratory evidence for HIV infection: 1) inclusion of HIV encephalopathy, HIV wasting syndrome, and a broader range of specific AIDS-indicative diseases (section II.A); 2) inclusion of AIDS patients whose indicator diseases are diagnosed presumptively (section II.B); and 3) elimination of exclusions due to other causes of immunodeficiency (section I.A.).

Application of the definition for children differs from that for adults in two ways. First, multiple or recurrent serious bacterial infections and lymphoid interstitial pneumonia/pulmonary lymphoid hyperplasia are accepted as indicative of AIDS among children but not among adults. Second, for children less than 15 months of age whose mothers are thought to have had HIV infection during the child's perinatal period, the laboratory criteria for HIV infection because of the persistence of passively acquired maternal antibodies less than 15 months after birth.

*Adapted from *Morbidity and Mortality Weekly Report.* Centers for Disease Control, Department of Health and Human Services, Vol 36, August 14, 1987. Used by permission.

The new definition is effective immediately. State and local health departments are requested to apply the new definition henceforth to patients reported to them. The initiation of the actual reporting of cases that meet the new definition is targeted for September 1, 1987, when modified computer software and report forms should be in place to accommodate the changes. CSTE has recommended retrospective application of the revised definition to patients already reported to health departments.

1987 Revision of Case Definition for AIDS for Surveillance Purposes

For national reporting, a case of AIDS is defined as an illness characterized by one or more of the following "indicator" diseases, depending on the status of laboratory evidence of HIV infection, as shown below.

I. Without Laboratory Evidence Regarding HIV Infection
    If laboratory tests for HIV were not performed or gave inconclusive results and the patient had no other cause of immunodeficiency listed in section I.A below, then any disease listed in section I.B indicates AIDS if it was diagnosed by a definitive method.
    A. Causes of immunodeficiency that disqualify diseases as indicators of AIDS in the absence of laboratory evidence for HIV infection
        1. High-dose or long-term systemic corticosteroid therapy or other immunosuppressive/cytotoic therapy less than three months before the onset of the indicator disease
        2. Any of the following disease diagnosed less than three months after diagnosis of the indicator disease: Hodgkin's disease, non-Hodgkin's lymphoma (other than primary brain lymphoma), lymphocytic leukemia, multiple myeloma, any other cancer of lymphoreticular or histiocytic tissue, or angioimmunoblastic lymphadenopathy
        3. A genetic (congenital) immunodeficiency syndrome or an acquired immunodeficiency syndrome atypical of HIV infection, such as one involving hypogammaglobulinemia
    B. Indicator diseases diagnosed definitively
        1. Candidiasis of the esophagus, trachea, bronchi, or lungs
        2. Cryptococcosis, extrapulmonary
        3. Cryptosporidiosis with diarrhea persisting greater than one month
        4. Cytomegalovirus disease of an organ other than liver, spleen or lymph nodes in a patient greater than one month of age
        5. Herpes simplex virus infection causing a mucocutaneous ulcer that persists longer than 1 month; or bronchitis, pneumonitis, or esophagitis for any duration affecting a patient greater than one month of age
        6. Kaposi's sarcoma affecting a patient less than 60 years of age
        7. Lymphoma of the brain (primary) affecting a patient less than 60 years of age

8. Lymphoid interstitial pneumonia and/or pulmonary lymphoid hyperplasia (LIP/PLH complex) affecting a child less than 13 years of age
9. Mycobacterium avium complex or *M. kansasii* disease, disseminated (at a site other than or in addition to lungs, skin, or cervical or hilar lymph nodes)
10. *Pneumocystis carinii* pneumonia
11. Progressive multifocal leukoencephalopathy
12. Toxoplasmosis of the brain affecting a patient greater than one month of age

II. With Laboratory Evidence for HIV Infection

Regardless of the presence of other causes of immunodeficiency (section I.A), in the presence of laboratory evidence for HIV infection, any disease listed above (section I.B) or below (section II.A or II.B) indicates a diagnosis of AIDS.

A. Indicator diseases diagnosed definitively
1. Bacterial infections, multiple or recurrent (any combination of at least two within a 2-year period), of the following types affecting a child less than 13 years of age: septicemia, pneumonia, meningitis, bone or joint infection, or abscess of an internal organ or body cavity (excluding otitis media or superficial (including pneumococcus), or other pyogenic bacteria
2. Coccidioidomycosis, disseminated (at a site other than or in addition to lungs or cervical or hilar lymph nodes)
3. HIV encephalopathy (also called "HIV dementia," "AIDS dementia," or "subacute encephalitis due to HIV")
4. Histoplasmosis, disseminated (at a site other than or in addition to lungs or cervical or hilar lymph nodes)
5. Isosporiasis with diarrhea persisting greater than one month
6. Kaposi's sarcoma at any age
7. Lymphoma of the brain (primary) at any age
8. Other non-Hodgkin's lymphoma of B-cell or unknown immunologic phenotype and the following histologic types:
   a. Small noncleaved lymphoma (either Burkitt or non-Burkitt type)
   b. Immunoblastic sarcoma (equivalent to any of the following, although not necessarily all in combination: immunoblastic lymphoma, large-cell lymphoma, diffuse histiocytic lymphoma, diffuse undifferentiated lymphoma, or high-grade lymphoma)

   Note: Lymphomas are not included here if they are of T-cell immunologic phenotype or their histologic type is not described or is described as "lymphocytic," "lymphoblastic," "small cleaved," or "plasmacytoid lymphocytic."
9. Any mycobacterial disease caused by mycobacteria other than *M. tuberculosis*, disseminated (at a site other than or in addition to lungs, skin, or cervical or hilar lymph nodes)

      10. Disease caused by *M. tuberculosis*, extrapulmonary (involving at least one site outside the lungs, regardless of whether there is concurrent pulmonary involvement)

      11. Salmonella (non-typhoid) septicemia, recurrent

      12. HIV wasting syndrome (emaciation, "slim disease")

  B. Indicator diseases diagnosed presumptively

III. With Laboratory Evidence Against HIV Infection

With laboratory test results negative for HIV infection, a diagnosis of AIDS for surveillance purposes is ruled out *unless*:

  A. All the other causes of immunodeficiency listed above in Section I.A. are excluded; AND

  B. The patient has had either:

      1. *Pneumocystis carinii* pneumonia diagnosed by a definitive method; OR

      2. a. Any of the other diseases indicative of AIDS listed above in section I.B. diagnosed by a definitive method; AND

          b. A T-helper/inducer (CD4) lymphocyte count 400/mm^3.

Commentary

The surveillance of severe disease associated with HIV infection remains an essential, though not the only, indicator of the course of the HIV epidemic. The number of AIDS cases and the relative distribution of cases by demographic, geographic, and behavioral risk variables are the oldest indices of the epidemic, which began in 1981 and for which data are available retrospectively back to 1978. The original surveillance case definition, based on then-available knowledge, provided useful epidemiologic data on severe HIV disease.[1] To ensure a reasonable predictive value for underlying immunodeficiency caused by what was then an unknown agent, the indicators of AIDS in the old case definition were restricted to particular opportunistic diseases diagnosed by reliable methods in patients without specific known causes of immunodeficiency. After HIV was discovered to be the cause of AIDS, however, and highly sensitive and specific HIV-antibody tests became available, the spectrum of manifestations of HIV infection became better defined, and classification systems for HIV infection were developed.[2-5] It became apparent that some progressive, seriously disabling, and even fatal conditions (e.g., encephalopathy, wasting syndrome) affecting a substantial number of HIV-infected patients were not subject to epidemiologic surveillance, as they were not included in the AIDS case definition. For reporting purposes, the revision adds to the definition most of those severe, noninfectious, noncancerous HIV-associated conditions that are categorized in the CDC clinical classification systems for HIV infection among adults and children.[4-5]

Another limitation of the old definition was that AIDS-indicative diseases are diagnosed presumptively (i.e., without confirmation by methods required by the old definition) in 10 to 15 percent of patients diagnosed with such diseases; thus, an appreciable proportion of AIDS cases were missed for reporting purposes.[6-7] This proportion may be increasing, which would compromise the old case definition's usefulness as a tool for monitoring trends. The revised case definition permits the reporting of these clinically diagnosed cases as long as there is laboratory evidence of HIV infection.

The effectiveness of the revision depends on how extensively HIV-antibody tests are used. Approximately one-third of AIDS patients in the United States have been from New York City and San Francisco, where, since 1985, less than 7 percent have been reported with HIV-antibody test results, compared with greater than 60 percent in other areas. The impact of the revision on the reported numbers of AIDS cases will also depend on the proportion of AIDS patients in whom indicator diseases are diagnosed presumptively rather than definitively. The use of presumptive diagnostic criteria varies geographically, being more common in certain rural areas and in urban areas with many indigent AIDS patients.

To avoid confusion about what should be reported to health departments, the term "AIDS" should refer only to conditions meeting the surveillance definition. This definition is intended only to provide consistent statistical data for public health purposes. Clinicians will not rely on this definition alone to diagnose serious disease caused by HIV infection in individual patients because there may be additional information that would lead to a more accurate diagnosis. For example, patients who are not reportable under the definition because they have either a negative HIV-antibody test, or in the presence of HIV antibody, an opportunistic disease not listed in the definition as an indicator of AIDS nonetheless may be diagnosed as having serious HIV disease on consideration of other clinical or laboratory characteristics of HIV infection or a history of exposure to HIV.

Conversely, the AIDS surveillance definition may rarely misclassify other patients as having serious HIV disease if they have no HIV-antibody test but have an AIDS-indicative disease with a background incidence unrelated to HIV infection, such as cryptococcal meningitis.

The diagnosis criteria accepted by the AIDS surveillance case definition should not be interpreted as the standard of good medical practice. Presumptive diagnoses are accepted in the definition because not to count them would be to ignore substantial mobility resulting from HIV infection. Likewise, the definition accepts a reactive screening test for HIV antibody without confirmation by a supplemental test because a repeatedly reactive screening test result, in combination with an indicator disease, is highly indicative of true HIV disease. For national surveillance purposes, the tiny proportion of possibly false-positive screening tests in persons with AIDS-indicative diseases is of little consequence. For the individual patient, however, a correct diagnosis is critically important. The use of supplemental tests is, therefore, strongly endorsed. An increase in the diagnostic use of HIV-antibody tests could improve both the quality of medical care and the function of the new case definition, as well as assist in providing counselling to prevent transmission of HIV.

References

1. World Health Organization (1986). Acquired immunodeficiency syndrome (AIDS): WHO/CDC case definition for AIDS. *WHO Weekly Epidemiology Record* 61:69-72.

2. Haverkos, H.W., Gottlieb, M.S., Killen, J.Y., et al. (1985). Classification of HTLV-III/LAV-related diseases (Letter). *Journal of Infectious Diseases,* 152: 1095.

3. Redfield, R.R., Wright, D.C., Tramont, E.C (1986). The Walter Reed staging classification of HTLV-III infection. *New England Journal of Medicine,* 314:131-132.

4. Centers for Disease Control (1986). Classification system for human T-lymphotropic virus type III/lymphadenopathy-associated virus infections. *Morbidity and Mortality Weekly Report,* 35:334-339.

5. Centers for Disease Control (1987). Classification system for human immunodeficiency virus (HIV) infection in children under 13 years of age. *Morbidity and Mortality Weekly Report,* 36:225-230, 235.

6. Hardy, A.M., Starcher, E.T., Morgan, W.M., et al. (1987). Review of death certificates to assess completeness of AIDS case reporting. *Public Health Report,* 102(4):386-391.

7. Starcher, E.T., Biel, J.K, Rivera-Castano, R., et al. (1987). The impact of presumptively diagnosed opportunistic infections and cancers on national reporting of AIDS (Abstract). Washington, DC: III International Conference on AIDS, June 1-5.

Laboratory Evidence for or Against HIV Infection

1. For Infection:

    When patient has disease consistent with AIDS:

    a. A serum specimen from a patient greater than 15 months of age, or from a child less than 15 months of age whose mother is not thought to have had HIV infection during the child's perinatal period, that is repeatedly reactive for HIV antibody by a screening test (e.g., enzyme-linked immunosorbent assay (ELISA), as long as subsequent HIV-antibody tests (e.g., Western blot, immunofluorescence assay), if done, are positive; OR

    b. A serum specimen from a child less than 15 months of age, whose mother is thought to have had HIV infection during the child's perinatal period, that is repeatedly reactive for HIV antibody by a screening test (e.g., ELISA), plus increased serum immunoglobulin levels and at least one of the following abnormal immunologic test results: reduced absolute lymphocyte count, depressed CD4 (T-helper) lymphocyte count, or decreased CD4/CD8 (helper/suppressor) ratio, as long as subsequent antibody tests (e.g., Western blot, immunofluorescence assay), if done, are positive;

OR
c. A positive test for HIV serum antigen; OR
d. A positive HIV culture confirmed by both reverse transcriptase detection and a specific HIV-antigen test or in situ hybridization using a nucleic acid probe; OR
e. A positive result on any other highly specific test for HIV 9, for example, nucleic acid probe of peripheral blood lymphocytes).

2. Against Infection A nonreactive screening test for serum antibody to HIV (e.g., ELISA) without a reactive or positive result on any other test for HIV infection (e.g., antibody, antigen, culture), if done.

3. Inconclusive (Neither For nor Against Infection)
a. A repeatedly reactive screening test for serum antibody to HIV (e.g., ELISA) followed by a negative or inconclusive supplemental test (e.g., Western blot, immunofluorescence assay) without a positive HIV culture or serum antigen test, if done; OR
b. A serum specimen from a child less than 15 months of age, whose mother is thought to have had HIV infection during the child's perinatal period, that is repeatedly reactive for HIV antibody by a screening test, even if positive by a supplemental test, without additional evidence for immunodeficiency as described above (in section 1.b) and without a positive HIV culture or serum antigen test, if done.

Definitive Diagnostic Methods for Diseases Indicative of AIDS

Diseases	Definitive Diagnostic Methods
Cryptosporidiosis Cytomegalovirus Isosporiasis Kaposi's sarcoma Lymphoma Lymphoid pneumonia *Pneumocystis carinii* pneumonia Progressive multifocal leukoencephalopathy Toxoplasmosis	Microscopy (histology or cytology) or hyperplasia
Candidiasis	Gross inspection by endoscopy or autopsy or by microscopy (histology or cytology) on a specimen obtained directly from the tissues affected (including scrapings from the mucosal surface), not from a culture
Coccidioidomycosis Cryptococcosis Herpes simplex virus Histoplasmosis	Microscopy (histology or cytology), culture, or detection of antigen in a specimen obtained directly from the tissues affected or a fluid from those tissues
Tuberculosis Other mycobacteriosis Salmonellosis Other bacterial infection	Culture
HIV encephalopathy* (dementia)	Clinical findings of disabling cognitive and/or motor dysfunction interfering with occupation or activities of daily living, or loss of behavioral developmental milestones affecting a child. Progressing over weeks to months, in the absence of a concurrent illness or condition other than HIV infection that could explain the findings. Methods to rule out such concurrent illnesses and conditions must include cerebrospinal fluid examination and either brain imaging (computed tomography or magnetic resonance) or autopsy.
HIV wasting syndrome*	Findings of profound involuntary weight loss greater than 10 percent of baseline body weight plus either chronic diarrhea (at least two loose stools per day for greater than 30 days) or chronic weakness and documented fever (for greater than 30 days, intermittent or constant) in the absence of a concurrent illness or condition other than HIV infection that could explain the findings (e.g., cancer, tuberculosis, cryptosporidiosis, or other specific enteritis)

*For HIV encephalopathy and HIV wasting syndrome, the methods of diagnosis described here are not truly definitive, but are sufficiently rigorous for surveillance purposes.

Suggested Guidelines for Presumptive Diagnosis of Diseases Indicative of AIDS

Diseases	Presumptive Diagnostic Criteria
Candidiasis of esophagus	a. Recent onset of retrosternal on swallowing; AND b. Oral candidiasis diagnosed by the gross appearance of white patches or plaques on an erythematous base or by the microscopic appearance of fungal mycelial filaments in an uncultured specimen scraped from the oral mucosa
Cytomegalovirus retinitis	A characteristic appearance on serial ophthalmoscopic examinations (e.g., discrete patches of retinal whitening with distinct borders, spreading in a centrifugal manner, following blood vessels, progressing over several months, frequently associated with retinal vasculitis, hemorrhage, and necrosis). Resolution of active disease leaves retinal scarring and atrophy with retinal pigment epithelial mottling.
Mycobacteriosis	Microscopy of a specimen from stool or normally sterile body fluids or tissue from a site other than lungs, skin, or cervical or hilar lymph nodes, showing acid-fast bacilli of a species not identified by culture.
Kaposi's sarcoma	A characteristic gross appearance of an erythematous or violaceous plaque-like lesion on skin or mucous membrane. (*Note*: Presumptive diagnosis of Kaposi's sarcoma should not be made by clinicians who have seen few cases of it.)
Lymphoid interstitial pneumonia	Bilateral reticulonodular interstitial pulmonary infiltrates present on chest x-ray for greater than two months with no pathogen identified and no response to antibiotic treatment.
Pneumocystis carinii pneumonia	a. A history of dyspnea on exertion or nonproductive cough of recent onset (within the past three months); AND b. Chest x-ray evidence of diffuse bilateral interstitial infiltrates or gallium scan evidence of diffuse bilateral pulmonary disease; AND c. Arterial blood gas analysis showing an arterial pox of less than 70mmHg or a low respiratory diffusing capacity (less than 80 percent of predicted values) or an increase in the alveolar-arterial oxygen tension gradient; AND d. No evidence of a bacterial pneumonia
Toxoplasmosis of the brain	a. Recent onset of a focal neurologic abnormality consistent with intracranial disease or a reduced level of consciousness; AND b. Brain imaging evidence of a legion having a mass effect (on computed tomography or nuclear magnetic resonance) or the radiographic appearance of which is enhanced by injection of contrast medium; AND c. Serum antibody to toxoplasmosis or successful response to therapy for toxoplasmosis

The Issue of Consent

A patient has legal rights concerning his treatment that have been recognized for generations. One of these is the right to be fully informed of, and consent to, any treatment or tests which a healthcare provider plans to use. This is known as the doctrine of informed consent. Health care providers must understand this legal doctrine in order to provide such information to their patients, and fully informed decisions can ultimately be made by the patients or their agents.

The concept of the health-care provider is an ever-expanding concept. Traditionally, a health-care provider has been a physician, a dentist or a nurse. However, this concept has grown to include home healthcare workers, occupational and physical therapists, social workers, or any number of others involved with the care of the patient, including family members (for the purpose of this chapter, "family" shall include any person who is important to the patient). Healthcare, itself, is a changing field, with the focus shifting from the treatment of illness and disease, to a new area of disease prevention.

The nature of the health-care provider—patient relationship is one of performance by the health-care provider, unless some other arrangement has been expressly agreed upon. It is a relationship imposed, it is not required, on the provider to conform to the accepted standards of knowledge, training, experience, skill, diligence and due care for the patient's well-being. It also imposes a duty of confidentiality, both by court decisions and statutes. Usually the health-care provider is seen as a fiduciary to whom the patient entrusts his secret.

Patients often expect that doctors, or other health care personnel, to cure all their problems. Presumably, the doctor can offer nothing more than a qualified medical opinion. Thus, an inherent conflict arises between patient expectations and the knowledge and treatment that a professional can actually deliver. The two will often coincide. However, at times they may differ from what they do not.

The number of malpractice suits against doctors, and others, is rapidly increasing. A patient who sues has a greater chance of success if the health-care provider failed fully to inform the patient of all of the options and treatments available, as well as the advantages and disadvantages of each option.

The Duty to Inform the Patient

Consent to Treatment

Since the time of the common law, it has been a general rule that a physician must give a patient enough information for them to make sound judgments concerning their own medical treatment. This is the patient's right to self-determination. It is his own basic position. To inform a patient fully could result in a patient consenting to the patient's consent, and subsequent lawsuits (usually based on negligence actions involving, in this case, were based on assault and battery.

Appendix B

Recommendations for Prevention of HIV Transmission in Health-Care Settings*

Introduction

HIV, the virus that causes AIDS, is transmitted through sexual contact and exposure to infected blood or blood components and perinatally from mother to neonate. HIV has been isolated from blood, semen, vaginal secretions, saliva, tears, breast milk, cerebrospinal fluid, amniotic fluid, and urine and is likely to be isolated from other body fluids, secretions, and excretions. However, epidemiologic evidence has implicated only blood, semen, vaginal secretions, and possibly breast milk in transmission.

The increasing prevalence of HIV increases the risk that health-care workers will be exposed to blood from patients infected with HIV, especially when blood and body fluid precautions are not followed for all patients. Thus, this document emphasizes the need for health-care workers to consider **all** patients as potentially infected with HIV and/or other blood-borne pathogens and to adhere rigorously to infection-control precautions for minimizing the risk of exposure to blood and body fluids of all patients.

The recommendations contained in this document consolidate and update CDC recommendations published earlier for preventing HIV transmission in health-care settings: precautions for clinical and laboratory staffs[1] and precautions for health-care workers and allied professionals[2]; recommendations for preventing HIV transmission in the workplace[3] and during invasive procedures[4]; recommendations for preventing possible transmission of HIV from tears[5]; and recommendations for providing dialysis treatment for HIV-infected patients[6]. These recommendations also update portions of the "Guideline for Isolation Precautions in Hospitals"[7] and reemphasize some of the recommendations contained in "Infection Control Practices for Dentistry"[8] The recommendations

---

*Reprinted from: *Morbidity and Mortality Weekly Report*, Centers for Disease Control, Department of Health and Human Services. Vol. 36, August 21, 1987.

contained in this document have been developed for use in health-care settings and emphasize the need to treat blood and other body fluids from **all** patients as potentially infective. These same prudent precautions also should be taken in other settings in which persons may be exposed to blood or other body fluids.

Definition of Health-Care Workers

Health-care workers are defined as persons, including students and trainees, whose activities involve contact with patients or with blood or other body fluids from patients in a health-care setting.

Health-Care Workers with AIDS

As of July 10, 1987, a total of 1,875 (5.8 percent) of 32,395 adults with AIDS, who had been reported to the CDC national surveillance system and for whom occupational information was available, reported being employed in a health-care or clinical laboratory setting. In comparison, 6.8 million persons—representing 5.6 percent of the U.S. labor force—were employed in health services. Of the health-care workers with AIDS, 95 percent have been reported to exhibit high-risk behavior; for the remaining 5 percent, the means of HIV acquisition was undetermined. Health-care workers with AIDS were significantly more likely than other workers to have an undetermined risk (5 percent vs. 3 percent, respectively). For both health-care workers and non-health-care workers with AIDS, the proportion with an undetermined risk has not increased since 1982.

AIDS patients initially reported as not belonging to recognized risk groups are investigated by state and local health departments to determine whether possible risk factors exist. Of all health-care workers with AIDS reported to CDC who were initially characterized as not having an identified risk and for whom follow-up information was available, 66 percent have been reclassified because risk factors were identified or because the patient was found not to meet the surveillance case definition for AIDS. Of the 87 health-care workers currently categorized as having no identifiable risk, information is incomplete on 16 (18 percent) because of death or refusal to be interviewed; 38 (44 percent) are still being investigated. The remaining 33 (38 percent) health-care workers were interviewed or had other follow-up information available. The occupations of these 33 health-care workers were as follows: five physicians (15 percent); three of whom were surgeons; one dentist (3 percent); three nurses (9 percent), nine nursing assistants (27 percent); seven housekeeping or maintenance workers (21 percent); three clinical laboratory technicians (95 percent); one therapist (3 percent); and four others who did not have contact with patients (12 percent). Although 15 of these 33 health-care workers reported parenteral and/or other non-needlestick exposure to blood or body fluids from patients in the ten years preceding their diagnosis of AIDS, none of these exposures involved a patient with AIDS or known HIV infection.

Risk to Health-Care Workers of Acquiring HIV in Health-Care Settings

Health-care workers with documented percutaneous or mucous-membrane exposures to blood or body fluids of HIV-infected patients have been prospectively evaluated to determine the risk of infection after such exposures. As of June 30, 1987, 883 health-care workers have been tested for antibody to HIV in an ongoing surveillance project conducted by CDC.[9] Of these, 708 (80 percent) had percutaneous exposures to blood, and 175 (20 percent) had a mucous membrane or an open wound contaminated by blood or body fluid. Of 396 health-care workers, each of whom had only a convalescent-phase serum sample obtained and tested greater than 90 days post-exposure, one—for whom heterosexual transmission could not be ruled out—was seropositive for HIV antibody. For 425 additional health-care workers, both acute- and convalescent-phase serum samples were obtained and tested; none of 74 health-care workers with non-percutaneous exposures seroconverted, and three (0.9 percent) of 351 with percutaneous exposures seroconverted. None of these three health-care workers had other documented risk factors for infection.

Two other prospective studies to assess the risk of nosocomial acquisition of HIV infection for health-care workers are ongoing in the United States. As of April 30, 1987, 332 health-care workers with a total of 453 needlestick or mucous membrane exposures to blood or other body fluids of HIV-infected patients were tested for HIV antibody at the National Institutes of Health[10] These exposed workers included 103 with needlestick injuries and 229 with mucous membrane exposures; none had seroconverted. A similar study at the University of California of 129 health-care workers with documented needlestick injuries or mucous membrane exposures to blood or other body fluids from patients with HIV infection has not identified any seroconversions.[11] Results of a prospective study in the United Kingdom identified no evidence of transmission among 150 health-care workers with parenteral or mucous membrane exposures to blood or other body fluids, secretions, or excretions from patients with HIV infection.[12]

In addition to health-care workers enrolled in prospective studies, eight persons who provided care to infected patients and denied other risk factors have been reported to have acquired HIV infection. Three of these health-care workers had needlestick exposures to blood from infected patients.[13-15] Two were persons who provided nursing care to infected persons; although neither sustained a needlestick injury; both had extensive contact with blood or other body fluids, and neither observed recommended barrier precautions.[16-17] The other three were health-care workers with non-needlestick exposures to blood from infected patients.[18] Although the exact route of transmission for these last three infections is not known, all three persons had direct contact of their skin with blood from infected patients, all had skin lesions that may have been contaminated by blood, and one also had a mucous membrane exposure.

A total of 1,231 dentists and hygienists, many of whom practiced in areas with many AIDS cases, participated in a study to determine the prevalence of antibody to HIV; one dentist (0.1 percent) had HIV antibody. Although no exposure to a known HIV-infected person could be documented, epidemiologic investigation did not identify any other risk factor for infection. The infected dentist, who had also had a history of sustaining needlestick injuries and trauma to his hands, did not routinely wear gloves when providing dental care.[19]

Precautions to Prevent Transmission of HIV

Universal Precautions

Since medical history and examination cannot reliably identify all patients infected with HIV or other blood-borne pathogens, blood and body-fluid precautions should be consistently used for **all** patients. This approach, previously recommended by CDC[3-4], and referred to as "universal blood and body-fluid precautions" or "universal precautions," should be used in the care of **all** patients, especially including those in emergency-care settings in which the risk of blood exposure is increased and the infection status of the patient is usually unknown.[20]

1. All health-care workers should routinely use appropriate barrier precautions to prevent skin and mucous membrane exposure when contact with blood or touching blood and body fluids, mucous membranes, or nonintact skin of all patients, for handling items or surfaces soiled with blood or body fluids, and for performing venipuncture and other vascular access procedures. Gloves should be changed after contact with each patient. Masks and protective eye wear or face shields should be worn during procedures that are likely to generate droplets of blood or other body fluids to prevent exposure of mucous membranes of the mouth, nose, and eyes. Gowns or aprons should be worn during procedures that are likely to generate splashes of blood or other body fluids.

2. Hands and other skin surfaces should be washed immediately and thoroughly if contaminated with blood or other body fluids. Hands should be washed immediately after gloves are removed.

3. All health-care workers should take precautions to prevent injuries caused by needles, scalpels, and other sharp instruments or devices during procedures; when cleaning used instruments; during disposal of used needles; and when handling sharp instruments after procedures. To prevent needlestick injuries, needles should not be recapped, purposely bent or broken by hand, removed from disposable syringes, or otherwise manipulated by hand. After they are used, disposable syringes and needles, scalpel blades, and other sharp items should be placed in puncture-resistant containers for disposal; the puncture-resistant containers should be located as close as practical to the use area. Large-bore reusable needles should be placed in a puncture-resistant container for transport to the reprocessing area.

4. Although saliva has not been implicated in HIV transmission, to minimize the need for emergency mouth-to-mouth resuscitation, mouthpieces, resuscita-

tion bags, or other ventilation devices should be available for use in areas in which the need for resuscitation is predictable.

5. Health-care workers who have exudative lesions or weeping dermatitis should refrain from all direct patient care and from handling patient-care equipment until the condition resolves.

6. Pregnant health-care workers are not known to be at greater risk of contracting HIV infection than health-care workers who are not pregnant; however, if a health-care worker develops HIV infection during pregnancy, the infant is at risk of infection resulting from perinatal transmission. Because of this risk, pregnant health-care workers should be especially familiar with and strictly adhere to precautions to minimize the risk of HIV transmission.

Implementation of universal blood and body-fluid precautions for **all** patients eliminates the need for use of the isolation category of "blood and body fluid precautions" previously recommended by CDC[7] for patients known or suspected to be infected with blood-borne pathogens. Isolation precautions (e.g., enteric, "AFB" [7]) should be used as necessary if associated conditions, such as infectious diarrhea or tuberculosis, are diagnosed or suspected.

Precautions for Invasive Procedures

In this document, an invasive procedure is defined as surgical entry into tissues, cavities, or organs or repair of major traumatic injuries 1) in an operating or delivery room, emergency department, or outpatient setting, including both physicians' and dentists offices; 2) cardiac catheterization and angiographic procedures; 3) a vaginal or cesarean delivery or other invasive obstetric procedure during which bleeding may occur; or 4) the manipulation, cutting, or removal of any oral or perioral tissues, including tooth structure, during which bleeding occurs or the potential for bleeding exists. The universal blood and body fluid precautions listed above, combined with the precautions listed below, should be the minimum precautions for **all** such invasive procedures.

1. All health-care workers who participate in invasive procedures must routinely use appropriate barrier precautions to prevent skin and mucous membrane contact with blood and other body fluids of all patients. Gloves and surgical masks must be worn for all invasive procedures. Protective eye wear or face shields should be worn for procedures that commonly result in the generation of droplets, splashing of blood or other body fluids, or the generation of bone chips. Gowns or aprons made of materials that provide an effective barrier should be worn during invasive procedures that are likely to result in the splashing of blood or other body fluids. All health-care workers who perform or assist in vaginal or cesarean deliveries should wear gloves and gowns when handling the placenta or the infant until blood and amniotic fluid have been removed from the infant's skin and should wear gloves during postdelivery care of the umbilical cord.

2. If a glove is torn or a needlestick or other injury occurs, the glove should be removed and a new glove used as promptly as patient safety permits; the needle or instrument involved in the incident should also be removed from the sterile field.

Precautions for Dentistry*

Blood, saliva, and gingival fluid from **all** dental patients should be considered infective. Special emphasis should be placed on the following precautions for preventing transmission of blood-borne pathogens in dental practice in both institutional and noninstitutional settings.

1. In addition to wearing gloves for contact with oral mucous membranes of all patients, all dental workers should wear surgical masks and protective eye wear or chin-length plastic face shields during dental procedures in which splashing or spattering of blood, saliva, or gingival fluids is likely. Rubber dams, high-speed evacuation, and proper patient positioning, when appropriate, should be utilized to minimize generation of droplets and spatter.

2. Handpieces should be sterilized after use with each patient, since blood, saliva, or gingival fluid of patients may be aspirated into the handpiece or waterline. Handpieces that cannot be sterilized should at least be flushed, the outside surface cleaned and wiped with a suitable chemical germicide, and then rinsed. Handpieces should be flushed at the beginning of the day and after use with each patient. Manufacturers' recommendations should be followed for use and maintenance of waterlines and check valves and for flushing of handpieces. The same precautions should be used for ultrasonic scalers and air/water syringes.

3. Blood and saliva should be thoroughly and carefully cleaned from material that has been used in the mouth (e.g., impression materials, bite registration), especially before polishing and grinding intraoral devices. Contaminated materials, impressions, and intraoral devices should also be cleaned and disinfected before being handled in the dental laboratory and before they are placed in the patient's mouth. Because of the increasing variety of dental materials used intraorally, dental workers should consult with manufacturers as to the stability of specific materials when using disinfection procedures.

4. Dental equipment and surfaces that are difficult to disinfect (e.g., light handles or x-ray unit heads) and that may become contaminated should be wrapped with impervious-backed paper, aluminum foil, or clear plastic wrap. The coverings should be removed and discarded, and clean coverings should be put in place after use with each patient.

Precautions for Autopsies or Morticians' Services

In addition to the universal blood and body-fluid precautions listed above, the following precautions should be used by persons performing postmortem procedures:

1. All persons performing or assisting in postmortem procedures should wear gloves, masks, protective eye wear, gowns, and waterproof aprons.

2. Instruments and surfaces contaminated during postmortem procedures should be decontaminated with an appropriate chemical germicide.

---

*General infection-control precautions are more specifically addressed in previous recommendations for infection-control practices for dentistry.[8]

Precautions for Dialysis

Patients with end-stage renal disease who are undergoing maintenance dialysis and who have HIV infection can be dialyzed in hospital-based or freestanding dialysis units using conventional infection control precautions.[21] Universal blood and body-fluid precautions should be used when dialyzing all patients.

Strategies for disinfecting the dialysis fluid pathways of the hemodialysis machine are targeted to control bacterial contamination and generally consist of using 500 to 750 parts per million (ppm) of sodium hypochlorite (household bleach) for 30 to 40 minutes or 1.5 to 2.0 percent formaldehyde overnight. In addition, several chemical germicides formulated to disinfect dialysis machines are commercially available. None of these protocols or procedures need to be changed for dialyzing patients infected with HIV.

Patients infected with HIV can be dialyzed by either hemodialysis or peritoneal dialysis and do not need to be isolated from other patients. The type of dialysis treatment (i.e., hemodialysis or peritoneal dialysis) should be based on the needs of the patient. The dialyzer may be discarded after each use. Alternatively, centers that reuse dialyzers—that is, a specific single-use dialyzer is issued to a specific patient, removed, cleaned, disinfected, and reused several times on the same patient only—may include HIV-infected patients in the dialyzer-reuse program. An individual dialyzer must never be used on more than one patient.

Precautions for Laboratories*

Blood and other body fluids from all patients should be considered infective. To supplement the universal blood and body-fluid precautions listed above, the following precautions are recommended for health-care workers in clinical laboratories.

1. All specimens of blood and body fluids should be put in a well-constructed container with a secure lid to prevent leaking during transport. Care should be taken when collecting each specimen to avoid contaminating the outside of the container and of the laboratory form accompanying the specimen.

2. All persons processing blood and body-fluid specimens (e.g., removing tops from vacuum tubes) should wear gloves. Masks and protective eye wear should be worn if mucous-membrane contact with blood or body fluids is anticipated. Gloves should be changed and hands washed after completion of specimen processing.

3. For routine procedures, such as histologic and pathologic studies or microbiologic culturing, a biological safety cabinet is not necessary. However, biological safety cabinets (Class I or II) should be used whenever procedures are conducted that have a high potential for generating droplets. These include activities such as blending, sonicating, and vigorous mixing.

4. Mechanical pipetting devices should be used for manipulating all liquids in the laboratory. Mouth pipetting must not be done.

5. Use of needles and syringes should be limited to situations in which there is no alternative, and the recommendations for preventing injuries with needles outlined under universal precautions should be followed.

---

*Additional precautions for research and industrial laboratories are addressed elsewhere.[22-23]

6. Laboratory work surfaces should be decontaminated with an appropriate chemical germicide after a spill of blood or other body fluids and when work activities are completed.
7. Contaminated materials used in laboratory tests should be decontaminated before reprocessing or be placed in bags and disposed of in accordance with institutional policies for disposal of infective waste.[24]
8. Scientific equipment that has been contaminated with blood or other body fluids should be decontaminated and cleaned before being repaired in the laboratory or transported to the manufacturer.
9. All persons should wash their hands after completing laboratory activities and should remove protective clothing before leaving the laboratory.

Implementation of universal blood and body-fluid precautions for **all** patients eliminates the need for warning labels on specimens since blood and other body fluids from all patients should be considered infective.

Environmental Considerations for HIV Transmission

No environmentally mediated mode of HIV transmission has been documented. Nevertheless, the precautions described below should be taken routinely in the care of **all** patients.

Sterilization and Disinfection

Standard sterilization and disinfection procedures for patient-care equipment currently recommended for use[25-26] in a variety of health-care settings—including hospitals, medical and dental clinics and offices, hemodialysis centers, emergency care facilities, and long-term nursing-care facilities—are adequate to sterilize or disinfect instruments, devices, or other items contaminated with blood or other body fluids from persons infected with blood-borne pathogens including HIV.[21,23]

Instruments or devices that enter sterile tissue or the vascular system of any patient or through which blood flows should be sterilized before reuse. Devices or items that contact intact mucous membranes should be sterilized or receive high-level disinfection, a procedure that kills vegetative organisms and viruses but not necessarily large numbers of bacterial spores. Chemical germicides that are registered with the U.S. Environmental Protection Agency (EPA) as "sterilants" may be used either for sterilization or for high-level disinfection depending on contact time.

Contact lenses used in trial fittings should be disinfected after each fitting by using a hydrogen peroxide contact lens disinfecting system, or, if compatible, with heat [78 C to 80 C (172.4 to 176.0 F)] for 10 minutes.

Medical devices or instruments that require sterilization or disinfection should be thoroughly cleaned before being exposed to the germicide, and the manufacturer's instructions for the use of the germicide should be followed. Further, it is important that the manufacturer's specifications for compatibility of the medical device with chemical germicides be closely followed. Information on specific label claims of commercial germicides can be obtained by writing to the

Disinfectants Branch, Office of Pesticides, Environmental Protection Agency, 401 M Street, SW, Washington, DC, 20460.

Studies have shown that HIV is inactivated rapidly after being exposed to commonly used chemical germicides at concentrations that are much lower than used in practice.[27-30] Embalming fluids are similar to the types of chemical germicides that have been tested and found to completely inactivate HIV. In addition to commercially available chemical germicides, a solution of sodium hypochlorite (household bleach) prepared daily is an inexpensive and effective germicide. Concentrations ranging from approximately 500 ppm (1:100 dilution of household bleach) sodium hypochlorite to 5,000 ppm (1:10 dilution of household bleach) are effective depending on the amount of organic material (e.g., blood, mucus) present on the surface to be cleaned and disinfected. Commercially available chemical germicides may be more compatible with certain medical devices that might be corroded by repeated exposure to sodium hypochlorite, especially to the 1:10 dilution.

Survival of HIV in the Environment

The most extensive study on the survival of HIV after drying involved greatly concentrated HIV samples, that is, 10 million tissue-culture infectious doses per milliliter (31). This concentration is at least 100,000 times greater than that typically found in the blood or serum of patients with HIV infection. HIV was detectable by tissue-culture techniques one to three days after drying, but the rate of inactivation was rapid. Studies performed at CDC have also shown that drying HIV causes a rapid (within several hours) 1 to 2 log (90 to 99 percent) reduction in HIV concentration. In tissue-culture fluid, cell-free HIV could be detected up to 15 days at room temperature, up to 11 days at 37C (98.6 F), and up to one day if the HIV was cell-associated.

When considered in the context of environmental conditions in health-care facilities, these results do not require any changes in currently recommended sterilization, disinfection, or housekeeping strategies. When medical devices are contaminated with blood or other body fluids, existing recommendations include the cleaning of these instruments, followed by disinfection or sterilization, depending on the type of medical device. These protocols assume "worst-case" conditions of extreme virologic and microbiologic contamination, and whether viruses have been inactivated after drying plays no role in formulating these strategies. Consequently, no changes in published procedures for cleaning, disinfecting, or sterilizing need to be made.

Housekeeping

Environmental surfaces such as walls, floors, and other surfaces are not associated with transmission of infections to patients or health-care workers. Therefore, extra-ordinary attempts to disinfect or sterilize these environmental surfaces are not necessary. However, cleaning and removal of soil should be done routinely.

Cleaning schedules and methods vary according to the area of the hospital or institution, type of surface to be cleaned, and the amount and type of soil present. Horizontal surfaces (e.g., bedside tables and hard-surfaced flooring) in patient-care areas are usually cleaned on a regular basis, when soiling or spills occur, and when a patient is discharged. Cleaning of walls, blinds, and curtains is recommended only if they are visibly soiled. Disinfectant fogging is an unsatisfactory method of decontaminating air and surfaces and is not recommended.

Disinfectant-detergent formulations registered by EPA can be used for cleaning environmental surfaces, but the actual physical removal of microorganisms by scrubbing is probably at least as important as any antimicrobial effect of the cleaning agent used. Therefore, cost, safety, and acceptability by housekeepers can be the main criteria for selecting any such registered agent. The manufacturers' instructions for appropriate use should be followed.

Cleaning and Decontaminating Spills of Blood or Other Body Fluids.

Chemical germicides that are approved for use as "hospital disinfectants" and are tuberculocidal when used at recommended dilutions can be used to decontaminate spills of blood and other body fluids. Strategies for decontaminating spills of blood and other body fluids in a patient-care setting are different than for spills of cultures or other materials in clinical, public health, or research laboratories. In patient-care areas, visible material should first be removed and then the area should be decontaminated. With large spills of cultured or concentrated infectious agents in the laboratory, the contaminated area should be flooded with a liquid germicide before cleaning, then decontaminated with fresh germicidal chemical. In both settings, gloves should be worn during the cleaning and decontaminating procedures.

Laundry.

Although soiled linen has been identified as a source of large numbers of certain pathogenic microorganisms, the risk of actual disease transmission is negligible. Rather than rigid procedures and specifications, hygienic and common-sense storage and processing of clean and soiled linen are recommended.[26] Soiled linen should be handled as little as possible and with minimum agitation to prevent gross microbial contamination of the air and of persons handling the linen. All soiled linen should be bagged at the location where it was used; it should not be sorted or rinsed in patient-care areas. Linen soiled with blood or body fluids should be placed and transported in bags that prevent leakage. If hot water is used, linen should be washed with detergent in water at least 71 C (160 F) for 25 minutes. If low-temperature [less than 70 C (158 F)], laundry cycles are used, chemicals suitable for low-temperature washing at proper use concentration should be used.

Infective Waste.

There is no epidemiologic evidence to suggest that most hospital waste is any more infective than residential waste. Moreover, there is no epidemiologic evidence that hospital waste has caused disease in the community as a result of improper disposal. Therefore, identifying wastes for which special precautions are indicated is largely a matter of judgment about the relative risk of disease transmission. The most practical approach to the management of infective waste is to identify those wastes with the potential for causing infection during handling and disposal and for which some special precautions appear prudent. Hospital wastes for which special precautions appear prudent include microbiology laboratory waste, pathology waste, and blood specimens or blood products. While any item that has had contact with blood, exudates. or secretions may be potentially infective, it is not usually considered practical or necessary to treat all such waste as infective.[23,26] Infective waste, in general, should either be incinerated or should be autoclaved before disposal in a sanitary landfill. Bulk blood, suctioned fluids, excretions, and secretions may be carefully poured down a drain connected to a sanitary sewer. Sanitary sewers may also be used to dispose of other infectious wastes capable of being ground and flushed into the sewer.

Implementation of Recommended Precautions

Employers of health-care workers should ensure that policies exist for:

1. Initial orientation and continuing education and training of all health-care workers—including students and trainees—on the epidemiology, modes of transmission, and prevention of HIV and other blood-borne infections and the need for routine use of universal blood and body-fluid precautions for **all** patients.
2. Provision of equipment and supplies necessary to minimize the risk of infection with HIV and other blood-borne pathogens.
3. Monitoring adherence to recommended precautions, counseling, education, and/or retraining should be provided, and, if necessary, appropriate disciplinary action should be considered.

Professional associations and labor organizations, through continuing education efforts, should emphasize the need for health-care workers to follow recommended precautions.

Serologic Testing for HIV Infection

Background

A person is identified as infected with HIV when a sequence of tests, starting with repeated enzyme immunoassays (EIA) and including a Western blot or similar, more specific assay, are repeatedly reactive. Persons infected with HIV usually develop antibody against the virus within 6 to 12 weeks after infection.

The sensitivity of the currently licensed EIA tests is at least 99 percent when they are performed under optimal laboratory conditions on serum specimens from persons infected for greater than 12 weeks. Optimal laboratory conditions include the use of reliable reagents, provision of continuing education of personnel, quality control of procedures, and participation in performance-evaluation programs. Given this performance, the probability of a false-negative test is remote except during the first several weeks after infection, before detectable antibody is present. The proportion of infected persons with a false-negative test attributed to absence of antibody in the early stages of infection is dependent on both the incidence and prevalence of HIV infection in a population.

The specificity of the currently licensed EIA tests is approximately 99 percent when repeatedly reactive tests are considered. Repeat testing of initially reactive specimens by EIA is required to reduce the likelihood of laboratory error. To increase further the specificity of serologic tests, laboratories must use a supplemental test, most often the Western blot, to validate repeatedly reactive EIA results. Under optimal laboratory conditions, the sensitivity of the Western blot test is comparable to or greater than that of a repeatedly reactive EIA, and the Western blot is highly specific when strict criteria are used to interpret the test results. The testing sequence of a repeatedly reactive EIA and a positive Western blot test is highly predictive of HIV infection, even in a population with a low prevalence of infection. If the Western blot test result is in determinant, the testing sequence is considered equivocal for HIV infection. When this occurs, the Western blot test should be repeated on the same serum sample, and, if still in determinant, the testing sequence should be repeated on a sample collected 3 to 6 months later. Use of other supplemental tests may aid in interpreting of results on samples that are persistently in determinant by Western blot.

Testing of Patients

Previous CDC recommendations have emphasized the value of HIV serologic testing of patients for 1) management of parenteral or mucous membrane exposures of health-care workers, 2) patient diagnosis and management, and 3) counseling and serologic testing to prevent and control HIV transmission in the community. In addition, more recent recommendations have stated that hospitals, in conjunction with state and local health departments, should periodically determine the prevalence of HIV infection among patients from age groups at highest risk of infection.[32]

Adherence to universal blood and body-fluid precautions recommended for the care of all patients will minimize the risk of transmission of HIV and other blood-borne pathogens from patients to health-care workers. The utility of routine HIV serologic testing of patients as an adjunct to universal precautions is unknown. Results of such testing may not be available in emergency or outpatient settings. In addition, some recently infected patients will not have detectable antibody to HIV.

Personnel in some hospitals have advocated serologic testing of patients in settings in which exposure of health-care workers to large amounts of patients' blood may be anticipated. Specific patients for whom serologic testing has been advocated include those undergoing major operative procedures and those undergoing treatment in critical care units, especially if they have conditions involving uncontrolled bleeding. Decisions regarding the need to establish testing programs for patients should be made by physicians or individual institutions. In addition, when deemed appropriate, testing of individual patients may be performed on agreement between the patient and the physician providing care.

In addition to the universal precautions recommended for all patients, certain additional precautions for the care of HIV-infected patients undergoing major surgical operations have been proposed by personnel in some hospitals. For example, surgical procedures on an HIV-infected patient might be altered so that hand-to-hand passing of sharp instruments would be eliminated; stapling instruments rather than hand-suturing equipment might be used to perform tissue approximation; electrocautery devices rather than scalpels might be used as cutting instruments; and, even though uncomfortable, gowns that totally prevent seepage of blood onto the skin of members of the operative team might be worn. While such modifications might further minimize the risk of HIV infection for members of the operative team, some of these techniques could result in prolongation of operative time and could potentially have an adverse effect on the patient.

Testing programs, if developed, should include the following principles:

● Obtaining consent for testing
● Informing patients of test results, and providing counseling for seropositive patients by properly trained persons
● Assuring that confidentiality safeguards are in place to limit knowledge of test results to those directly involved in the care of infected patients or as required by law
● Assuring that identification of infected patients will not result in denial of needed care or provision of suboptimal care
● Evaluating prospectively 1) the efficacy of the program in reducing the incidence of parenteral, mucous-membrane, or significant cutaneous exposures of health-care workers to the blood or other body fluids of HIV-infected patients and 2) the effect of modified procedures on patients.

Testing of Health-Care Workers

Although transmission of HIV from infected health-care workers to patients has not been reported, transmission during invasive procedures remains a possibility. Transmission of HBV—a blood-borne agent with a considerably greater potential for nosocomial spread—from health-care workers to patients has been documented. Such transmission has occurred in situations (e.g., oral and gynecologic surgery) in which health-care workers, when tested, had very high concentrations of HBV in their blood (at least 100 million infectious virus particles per milliliter, a concentration much higher than occurs with HIV infection), and the health-care workers sustained a puncture wound while performing invasive procedures or had exudative or weeping lesions or microlacerations that allowed virus to contaminate instruments or open wounds of patients.[33-34]

The hepatitis B experience indicates that only those health-care workers who perform certain types of invasive procedures have transmitted HBV to patients. Adherence to recommendations in this document will minimize the risk of transmission of HIV and other blood-borne pathogens from health-care workers to patients during invasive procedures. Since transmission to their patients has not been reported and would be expected to occur only very rarely, if at all, the utility of routine testing of such health care workers who perform invasive procedures, the frequency of testing, as well as the issues of consent, confidentiality, and consequences of test results—as previously outlined for testing programs for patients—must be addressed.

Management of Infected Health-Care Workers

Health-care workers with impaired immune systems resulting from HIV infection or other causes are at increased risk of acquiring or experiencing serious complications of infectious disease. Of particular concern is the risk of severe infection following exposure to patients with infectious diseases that are easily transmitted if appropriate precautions are not taken (e.g., measles, varicella). Any health-care worker with an impaired immune system should be counseled about the potential risk associated with taking care of patients with any transmissible infection and should continue to follow existing recommendations for infection control to minimize risk of exposure to other infectious agents.[7,35] Recommendations of the Immunization Practices Advisory Committee (ACIP) and institutional policies concerning requirements for vaccinating health-care workers with live-virus vaccines (e.g., measles, rubella) should also be considered.

The question of whether workers infected with HIV—especially those who perform invasive procedures—can adequately and safely be allowed to perform patient-care duties or whether their work assignments should be changed must be determined on an individual basis. These decisions should be made by the health-care worker's personal physician(s) in conjunction with the medical directors and personnel health service staff of the employing institution or hospital.

Management of Exposures

If a health-care worker has a parenteral (e.g., needlestick or cut) or mucous membrane (e.g., splash to the eye or mouth) exposure to blood or other body fluids or has a cutaneous exposure involving large amounts of blood or prolonged contact with blood—especially when the exposed skin is chapped, abraded, or afflicted with dermatitis—the source patient should be informed of the incident and tested for serologic evidence of HIV infection after consent is obtained. Policies should be developed for testing source patients in situations in which consent cannot be obtained (e.g., an unconscious patient).

If the source patient has AIDS, is positive for HIV antibody, or refuses the test, the health-care worker should be counseled regarding the risk of infection and evaluated clinically and serologically for evidence of HIV infection as soon as possible after the exposure. The health-care worker should be advised to report and seek medical evaluation for any acute febrile illness that occurs within 12 weeks after the exposure. Such an illness —particularly one characterized by fever, rash, or lymphadenopathy—may be indicative of recent HIV infection. Seronegative health-care workers should be retested 6 weeks post-exposure and on a periodic basis thereafter (e.g., 12 weeks and 6 months after exposure) to determine whether transmission has occurred. During this follow-up period— especially the first 6 to 12 weeks after exposure, when most infected persons are expected to seroconvert—exposed health-care workers should follow U.S. Public Health Service (PHS) recommendations for preventing transmission of HIV.[36-37]

No further follow-up of a health-care worker exposed to infection as described above is necessary if the source patient is seronegative unless the source patient is at high risk of HIV infection. In the latter case, a subsequent specimen (e.g., 12 weeks following exposure) may be obtained from the health-care worker for antibody testing. If the source patient cannot be identified, decisions regarding appropriate follow-up should be individualized. Serologic testing should be available to all health-care workers who are concerned that they may have been infected with HIV.

If a patient has a parenteral or mucous membrane exposure to blood or other body fluid of a health-care worker, the patient should be informed of the incident, and the same procedure outlined above for management of exposures should be followed for both the source health-care worker and the exposed patient.

References

1. Centers for Disease Control (1982). Acquired immunodeficiency syndrome (AIDS): Precautions for clinical and laboratory staffs. *Morbidity and Mortality Weekly Report,* 31: 577-580.

2. Centers for Disease Control (1983). Acquired immunodeficiency syndrome (AIDS): Precautions for health-care workers and allied professionals. *Morbidity and Mortality Weekly Report,* 32: 450-451.

3. Centers for Disease Control (1985). Recommendations for preventing transmission of infection with human T-lymphotropic virus type III/ lymphadenopathy-associated virus in the workplace. *Morbidity and Mortality Weekly Report,* 34: 681-686, 691-695.

4. Centers for Disease Control (1986). Recommendations for preventing transmission of infection with human T-lymphotropic virus type III/ lymphadenopathy-associated virus during invasive procedures. *Morbidity and Mortality Weekly Report,* 35: 221-223.

5. Centers for Disease Control (1985). Recommendations for preventing possible transmission of human T-lymphotropic virus type III/lymphadeno-pathy-associated virus from tears. *Morbidity and Mortality Weekly Report,* 34: 533-534.

6. Centers for Disease Control (1986). Recommendations for providing dialysis treatment to patients infected with human T-lymphotropic virus type III/lymphadenopathy-associated virus infection. *Morbidity and Mortality Weekly Report,* 35: 376-378, 383.

7. Garner, J.S. and Simmons, B.P. (1983). Guideline for isolation precautions in hospitals. *Infection Control,* 4 (suppl): 245-325.

8. Centers for Disease Control (1986). Recommended infection control practices for dentistry. *Morbidity and Mortality Weekly Report,* 35: 237-242.

9. McCray, E. (1986). The Cooperative Needlestick Surveillance Group. Occupational risk of the acquired immunodeficiency syndrome among health care workers. *New England Journal of Medicine,* 314: 1127-1132.

10. Henderson, D.K., Saah, A.J., Zak, B.J., et al. (1986). Risk of nosocomial infection with human T-cell lymphotropic virus type III/lymphadenopathy-associated virus in a large cohort of intensively exposed health care workers. *Annals of Internal Medicine,* 104: 644-647.

11. Gerberding, J.L., Bryant-LeBlanc, C.E., Nelson, K., et al. (1987). Risk of

transmitting the human immunodeficiency virus, cytomegalovirus, and hepatitis B virus to health care workers exposed to patients with AIDS and AIDS-related conditions. *Journal of Infectious Disease,* 156: 1-8.

12. McEvoy, M., Porter, K., Mortimer, P., et al. (1987). Prospective study of clinical, laboratory, and ancillary staff with accidental exposures to blood or other body fluids from patients infected with HIV. *British Medical Journal,* 294: 1595-1597.

13. Anonymous (1984). Needlestick transmission of HTLV-III from a patient infected in Africa. *Lancet,* 2: 1376-1377.

14. Oksenhendler, E., Harzic, M., LeRoux, J.M., et al. (1986). HIV infection with seroconversion after a superficial needlestick injury to the finger. *New England Journal of Medicine,* 315: 582.

15. Neisson-Vernant, C., Arfi, S., Mathez, D., et al. (1986). Needlestick HIV seroconversion in a nurse. *Lancet,* 2: 814.

16. Grint, P. and McEvoy, M. (1985). Two associated cases of the acquired immune deficiency syndrome (AIDS). *Public Health Laboratory Service Communicable Disease Surveillance Centre Report,* 42: 4.

17. Centers for Disease Control (1986). Apparent transmission of human T-lymphotropic virus type III/lymphadenopathy-associated virus from a child to a mother providing health care. *Morbidity and Mortality Weekly Report,* 35: 76-79.

18. Centers for Disease Control (1987). Update: Human immunodeficiency virus infections in health-care workers exposed to blood of infected patients. *Morbidity and Mortality Weekly Report,* 36: 285-289.

19. Kline, R.S., Phelan, J., Friedland, G.H., et al. (1985). Low occupational risk for HIV infection for dental professionals (Abstract). In Abstracts from the III International Conference on AIDS, Washington, DC, June 1-5.

20. Baker, J.L., Kelen, G.D., Sivertson, K.T., et al. (1987). Unsuspected human immunodeficiency virus in critically ill emergency patients. *Journal of American Medical Association,* 257: 2609-2611.

21. Favero, M.S. (1985). Dialysis-associated diseases and their control. In: Bennett, J.V. and Brachman, P.S. (Eds.), *Hospital Infections.* Boston: Little, Brown, pp 267-284.

22. Richardson, J.H. and Barkley, W.E. (Eds.) (1984). *Biosafety in Microbiological and Biomedical Laboratories.* Washington, DC: U.S. Department of Health and Human Services, Public Health Service. HHS Publication no. (CDC) 84-8395.

23. Centers for Disease Control (1986). Human T-lymphotropic virus type III/lymphadenopathy-associated virus: Agent summary statement. *Morbidity and Mortality Weekly Report,* 35: 540-542, 547-549.

24. Environmental Protection Agency (1986). *EPA guide for infectious waste management.* Washington, DC: Environmental Protection Agency, Publication no. EPA/530-SW-86-014.

25. Favero, M.S. Sterilization, disinfection, and antisepsis in the hospital. In

Manual of Clinical Microbiology, 4th ed. Washington, DC: American Society for Microbiology, HHS Publication no. 99-1117.

26. Garner, J.S. and Favero, M.S. (1985). *Guideline for Handwashing and Hospital Environmental Control*. Atlanta, GA: Public Health Service, Centers for Disease Control. HHS Publication no. 99-1117.

27. Spire, B., Montagnier, L., Barre-Sinoussi, F., et al. (1984). Inactivation of lymphadenopathy associated virus by chemical disinfectants. *Lancet*, 2: 899-901.

28. Martin, L.S., McDougal, J.S. and Loskoski, S.L. Disinfection and inactivation of the human T lymphotropic virus type III/lymphadenopathy-associated virus. *Journal of Infectious Disease*, 152: 400-403.

29. McDougal, J.S., Martin, L.S., Cort, S.P., et al. (1985). Thermal inactivation of the acquired immunodeficiency syndrome virus-III/lymphadenopathy-associated virus, with special reference to antihemophilic factor. *Journal of Clinical Investigation*, 76: 875-877.

30. Spire, B., Barre-Sinoussi, F., Dormont, D., et al. (1985). Inactivation of lymphadenopathy-associated virus by heat, gamma rays, and ultraviolet light. *Lancet*, 1: 188-189.

31. Resnik, L., Veren, K., Salahuddin, S.Z., et al. (1986). Stability and inactivation of HTLV-III/LAV under clinical and laboratory environments. *Journal of the American Medical Association*, 255: 1887-1891.

32. Centers for Disease Control. (1987). Public Health Service (PHS) guidelines for counseling and antibody testing to prevent HIV infection and AIDS. *Morbidity and Mortality Weekly Report*, 3: 509-515.

33. Kane, M.A. and Lettau, L.A. (1985). Transmission of HBV from dental personnel to patients. *Journal of the American Dental Association*, 110: 634-636.

34. Lettau, L.A., Smith, J.D., Williams, D., et al. (1986). Transmission of hepatitis B with resultant restriction of surgical practice. *Journal of the American Medical Association*, 255: 934-937.

35. Williams, W.W. (1983) Guideline for infection control in hospital personnel. *Infection Control*, 4 (suppl): 326-349.

36. Centers for Disease Control (1983). Prevention of acquired immunodeficiency syndrome (AIDS): Report of inter-agency recommendations. *Morbidity and Mortality Weekly Report*, 32: 101-103.

37. Centers for Disease Control (1985). Provisional Public Health Service inter-agency recommendations for screening donated blood and plasma for antibody to the virus causing acquired immunodeficiency syndrome. *Morbidity and Mortality Weekly Report*, 34: 1-5.

Appendix C

Perspectives in Disease Prevention and Health Promotion

Update: Universal Precautions for Prevention of Transmission of Human Immunodeficiency Virus, Hepatitis B Virus, and Other Bloodborne Pathogens in Health-Care Settings*

Introduction

The purpose of this report is to clarify and supplement the CDC publication entitled "Recommendations for prevention of HIV transmission in health-care settings."[†]

In 1983, CDC published a document entitled, "Guideline for isolation precautions in hospitals"[2] that contained a section entitled "Blood and body fluid precautions." The recommendations in this section called for blood and body fluid precautions when a patient was known or suspected to be infected with blood-borne pathogens. In August 1987, CDC published a document entitled "Recommendations for prevention of HIV transmission in health-care settings."[1] In contrast to the 1983 document, the 1987 document recommended that blood and body fluid precautions be consistently used for all patients regardless of their blood-borne infection status. This extension of blood and body fluid precautions to **all** patients is referred to as "universal blood and body fluid precautions" or "universal precautions." Under universal precautions, blood and certain body fluids of all patients are considered potentially infectious for HIV, HBV, and other blood-borne pathogens. Universal precautions are intended to prevent parenteral, mucous membrane, and non-intact skin exposures of health-care workers to blood-borne pathogens. In addition, immunization with HVB vaccine is recommended as an important adjunct to universal precautions for health-care workers who have exposures to blood.[3-4]

---

*Reprinted from *Morbidity and Mortality Weekly Report*. Centers for Disease Control, Department of Health and Human Services. Vol. 37:24, June 24, 1988. Used with permission.

†The August 1987 publication should be consulted for general information and specific recommendations not addressed in this update.

Since the recommendations for universal precautions were published in August 1987, CDC and the Food and Drug Administration (FDA) have received requests for clarification of the following issues: 1) body fluids to which universal precautions apply, 2) use of protective barriers, 3) use of gloves for phlebotomy, 4) selection of gloves for use while observing universal precautions, and 5) need for making changes in waste management programs as a result of adopting universal precautions.

Body Fluids to Which Universal Precautions Apply

Universal precautions apply to blood and to other body fluids containing visible blood. Occupational transmission of HIV and HBV to health-care workers by blood is documented.[4-5] Blood is the single most important source of HIV, HBV, and other blood borne pathogens in the occupational setting. Infection control efforts for HIV, HBV, and other blood-borne pathogens must focus on preventing exposures to blood as well as on delivery of HBV Immunization.

Universal precautions also apply to semen and vaginal secretions. Although both of these fluids have been implicated in the sexual transmission of HIV and HBV, they have not been implicated in occupational transmission from patient to health-care worker. This observation is not unexpected, since exposure to semen in the usual health-care setting is limited, and the routine practice of wearing gloves for performing vaginal examinations protects health-care workers from exposure to potentially infectious vaginal secretions.

Universal precautions also apply to tissues and to the following fluids: cerebrospinal fluid (CSF), synovial fluid, pleural fluid, peritoneal fluid, pericardial fluid, pericardial fluid, and amniotic fluid. The risk of transmission of HIV and HBV from these fluids is unknown; epidemiologic studies in the health-care and community setting are currently inadequate to assess the potential risk to health-care workers from occupational exposures to them. However, HIV has been isolated from CSF, synovial, and amniotic fluid[6-8], and HBsAg has been detected in synovial fluid, amniotic fluid, and peritoneal fluid.[9-11] One case of HIV transmission was reported after a percutaneous exposure to blood pleural fluid obtained by needle aspiration.[12] Whereas aseptic procedures used to obtain these fluids for diagnostic or therapeutic purposes protect health-care workers from skin exposures, they cannot prevent penetrating injuries due to contaminated needles or other sharp instruments.

Body Fluids to Which Universal Precautions Do Not Apply

Universal precautions do not apply to feces, nasal secretions, sputum, sweat, tears, urine, and vomitus unless they contain visible blood. The risk of transmission of HIV and HBV from these fluids and materials is extremely low or nonexistent. HIV has been isolated and HBsAg has been demonstrated in some of these fluids; however, epidemiologic studies in the health-care and community setting have not implicated these fluids or materials in the transmission of HIV and HBV infections.[13-14] Some of the above fluids and excretions represent a potential source for nosocomial and community-acquired infections with other pathogens, and recommendations for preventing the transmission of non-blood-borne pathogens have been published.[2]

Precautions for Other Body Fluids in Special Settings

Human breast milk has been implicated in perinatal transmission of HIV, and HBsAg has been found in the milk of mothers infected with HBV.[10,13] However, occupational exposure to human breast milk has not been implicated in the transmission of HIV nor HBV infection to health-care workers. Moreover, the health-care worker will not have the same type of intensive exposure to breast milk as the nursing neonate. Whereas universal precautions do not apply to human breast milk, gloves may be worn by health-care workers in situations where exposures to breast milk might be frequent, for example, in breast milk banking.

Saliva of some persons infected with HBV has been shown to contain HBV-DNA at concentrations of $1 = 1,000$ to $1 = 10,000$ of that found in the infected persons' serum.[15] HBsAg-positive saliva has been shown to be infectious when injected into experimental animals and in human bite exposures.[16-18] However, HBsAg-positive saliva has not been shown to be infectious when applied to oral mucous membranes in experimental primate studies[18] or through contamination of musical instruments or cardiopulmonary resuscitation dummies used by HBV carriers.[19,20] Epidemiologic studies of nonsexual household contacts of HIV-infected patients, including several small series in which HIV transmission failed to occur after bites or after percutaneous inoculation or contamination of cuts and open wounds with saliva from HIV-infected patients, suggest that the potential for salivary transmission of HIV is remote.[5,13,14,21,22] One case report from Germany has suggested the possibility of transmission of HIV in a household setting from an infected child to a sibling through a human bite.[23] The bite did not break the skin or result in bleeding. Since the date of seroconversion to HIV was not known for either child in this case, evidence for the role of saliva in the transmission of HIV from husband to wife by contact suggested the possibility of transmission of HIV from husband to wife by contact with saliva during kissing.[24] However, follow-up studies did not confirm HIV infection in the wife.[21]

Universal precautions do not apply to saliva. General infection control practices already in existence—including the use of gloves for digital examination of mucous membranes and endotracheal suctioning, and handwashing after exposure to saliva—should further minimize the minute risk, if any, for salivary transmission of HIV and HBV.[1,25] Gloves need not be worn when feeding patients and when wiping saliva from skin.

Special precautions, however, are recommended for dentistry.[1] Occupationally acquired infection with HBV in dental workers has been documented,[4] and two possible cases of occupationally acquired HIV infection involving dentists have been reported.[5,26] During dental procedures, contamination of saliva with blood is predictable, trauma to health care workers' hands is common, and blood spattering may occur. Infection control precautions for dentistry minimize the potential for non intact skin and mucous membrane contact of dental health-care workers to blood-contaminated saliva of patients. In addition, the use of gloves for oral examinations and treatment in the dental setting may also protect the patient's oral mucous membranes from exposures to blood, which may occur from breaks in the skin of dental workers' hands.

Use of Protective Barriers

Protective barriers reduce the risk of exposure of the health-care worker's skin or mucous membranes to potentially infective materials. For universal precautions, protective barriers reduce the risk of exposure to blood, body fluids containing visible blood, and other fluids to which universal precautions apply. Examples of protective barriers include gloves, gowns, masks, and protective eye wear. Gloves should reduce the incidence of contamination of hands, but they cannot prevent penetrating injuries due to needles or other sharp instruments. Masks and protective eye wear or face shields should reduce the incidence of contamination of mucous membranes of the mouth, nose, and eyes.

Universal precautions are intended to supplement rather than replace recommendations for routine infection control, such as handwashing and using gloves to prevent gross microbial contamination of hands.[27] Because specifying the types of barriers needed for every possible clinical situation is impractical, some judgment must be exercised.

The risk of nosocomial transmission of HIV, HBV, and other blood borne pathogens can be minimized if health-care workers use the following general guidelines.

1. Take care to prevent injuries when using needles, scalpels, and other sharp instruments or devices; when handling sharp instruments after procedures; when cleaning used instruments; and when disposing of used needles. Do not recap used needles by hand; do not remove used needles from disposable syringes and needles, scalpel blades, and other sharp items in puncture-resistant containers for disposal. Locate the puncture-resistant containers as close to the use area as is practical.
2. Use protective barriers to prevent exposure to blood, body fluids containing visible blood, and other fluids to which universal precautions apply. The type of protective barrier(s) should be appropriate for the procedure being performed and the type of exposure anticipated.
3. Immediately and thoroughly wash hands and other skin surfaces that are contaminated with blood, body fluids containing visible blood, or other body fluids to which universal precautions apply.

Glove Use for Phlebotomy

Gloves should reduce the incidence of blood contamination of hands during phlebotomy (drawing blood samples), but they cannot prevent penetrating injuries caused by needles or sharp instruments. The likelihood of hand contamination with blood containing HIV, HBV, or other blood-borne pathogens during phlebotomy depends on several factors: 1) the skill and technique of the health-care worker; 2) the frequency with which the health-care worker performs the procedure (other factors being equal, the cumulative risk of blood exposure is higher for a health-care worker who performs more procedures); 3) whether the procedure occurs in a routine or emergency situation (where blood contact may be more likely); and 4) the prevalence of infection with blood-borne pathogens in the patient population. The likelihood of infection after skin exposure to blood containing HIV or HBV depends on the concentration of virus (viral concentration is much higher for hepatitis B than for HIV), the duration of contact, the presence of skin lesions on the hands of the health-care workers, and—for HBV—the immune status of the health-care worker. Although not accurately quantified, the risk of HIV infection following intact skin contact with infective blood is certainly much less than the 0.5 percent risk following percutaneous needlestick exposures.[5] In universal precautions, *all* blood is assumed to be potentially infective for blood-borne pathogens, but in certain settings (e.g., volunteer blood donation centers) the prevalence of infection with some blood-borne pathogens (e.g., HIV, HBV) is known to be very low. Some institutions have relaxed recommendations for using gloves for phlebotomy procedures by skilled phlebotomists in settings where the prevalence of blood borne pathogens is known to be very low.

Institutions that judge that routine gloving for all phlebotomies is not necessary should periodically reevaluate their policy. Gloves should always be available to health-care workers who wish to use them for phlebotomy. In addition, the following general guidelines apply:

1. Use gloves for performing phlebotomy when the health-care worker has cuts, scratches, or other breaks in his skin.
2. Use gloves in situations where the health-care worker judges that hand contamination with blood may occur, for example, when performing phlebotomy on an uncooperative patient.
3. Use gloves for performing finger and/or heel sticks on infants and children.
4. Use gloves when persons are receiving training in phlebotomy.

Selection of Gloves

The Center for Devices and Radiological Health, FDA, has responsibility for regulating the medical glove industry. Medical gloves include those marketed as sterile surgical or non sterile examination gloves made of vinyl or latex. General purpose utility ("rubber") gloves are also used in the health-care setting, but they are not regulated by FDA since they are not promoted for medical use. There are no reported differences in barrier effectiveness between intact latex and intact vinyl used to manufacture gloves. Thus, the type of gloves selected should be appropriate for the task being performed.

The following general guidelines are recommended:

1. Use sterile gloves for procedures involving contact with normally sterile areas of the body.
2. Use examination gloves for procedures involving contact with mucous

membranes, unless otherwise indicated, and for other patient care or diagnostic procedures that do not require the use of sterile gloves.
3. Change gloves between patient contacts.
4. Do not wash or disinfect surgical or examination gloves for reuse. Washing with surfactants may cause "wicking," that is, the enhanced penetration of liquids through undetected holes in the glove. Disinfecting agents may cause deterioration.
5. Use general-purpose utility gloves (e.g., rubber household gloves) for housekeeping chores involving potential blood contact and for instrument cleaning and decontamination procedures. Utility gloves may be decontaminated and reused, but should be discarded if they are peeling, cracked, or discolored, or if they have punctures, tears, or other evidence of deterioration.

Waste Management

Universal precautions are not intended to change waste management programs previously recommended by CDC for health-care settings.[1] Policies for defining, collecting, storing, decontaminating, and disposing of infective waste are generally determined by institutions in accordance with state and local regulations. Information regarding waste management regulations in health-care settings may be obtained from state or local health departments or agencies responsible for waste management. Reported by: Center for Devices and Radiological Health, Food and Drug Administration. Hospital Infections Program, AIDS Program, and Hepatitis Branch, Division of Viral Diseases, Center for Infectious Diseases, National Institute for Occupational Safety and Health, Continuing Education Committee (CEC).

Editorial Note: Implementation of universal precautions does not eliminate the need for other category- or disease-specific isolation precautions, such as enteric precautions for infectious diarrhea or isolation for pulmonary tuberculosis.[1-2] In addition to universal precautions, detailed precautions have been developed for the following procedures and/or settings in which prolonged or intensive exposures to blood occur: invasive procedures, dentistry, autopsies or morticians' services, dialysis, and the clinical laboratory. These detailed precautions are found in the August 21, 1987 "Recommendations for prevention of HIV transmission in health-care settings."[1] In addition, specific precautions have been developed for research laboratories.[28]

References
1. Centers for Disease Control (1987). Recommendations for prevention of HIV transmission in health-care settings. *Mobility and Mortality Weekly Report*, 36(suppl 2S):229, 234, 239.
2. Garner, J.S. and Simmons, B.P. (1983). Guideline for isolation precautions in hospitals. *Infection Control*, 4:245-325.
3. Immunization Practices Advisory Committee (1985). Recommendations for protection against viral hepatitis. *Mobility and Mortality Weekly Report*, 34:313-324, 329-335.

4. Department of Labor, Department of Health and Human Services (1987). *Joint Advisory Notice: Protection Against Occupational Exposure to Hepatitis B Virus (HBV) and Human Immunodeficiency Virus (HIV).* Washington, DC: US Department of Labor, US Department of Health and Human Services.

5. Centers for Disease Control (1988). Update: Acquired immunodeficiency syndrome and human immunodeficiency virus infection among health-care workers. *Mobility and Mortality Weekly Report,* 37:229-234, 239.

6. Hollander, H. and Levy, J.A. (1987). Neurologic abnormalities and recovery of human immunodeficiency virus from cerebrospinal fluid. *Annuals Internal Medicine,* 106:692-695.

7. Wirthrington, R.H., Cornes, P., Harris, JRW, et al. (1987) Isolation of human immunodeficiency from synovial fluid of a patient with reactive arthritis. *British Medical Journal,* 294:484.

8. Mundy, D.C., Schinazi, R.F., Gerber, A.R., et al. (1987). Human immunodeficiency virus isolated from amniotic fluid. *Lancet,* 2:459-460.

9. Onion, D.K., Crumpacker, C.S. and Gilliland, B.C. (1971). Arthritis of hepatitis associated with Australia antigen. *Annals of Internal Medicine,* 75:29-33.

10. Lee, A.K.Y., Ip, H.M.H. and Wong, V.C.W. (1978). Mechanisms of maternal-fetal transmission of hepatitis B virus. *Journal of Infectious Diseases,* 138:668-671.

11. Bond, W.W., Petersen, N.J., Gravelle, C.R., et al. (1982). Hepatitis B virus in peritoneal dialysis fluid: A potential hazard. *Dialysis and Transplantation,* 11:592-600.

12. Oskenhendler, E., Harzic, M., LeRoux, J.-M., et al. (1986). HIV infection with seroconversion after a superficial needlestick injury to the finger (Letter). *New England Journal of Medicine,* 315:582.

13. Lifson, A.R. (1988). Do alternate modes for transmission of human immunodeficiency virus exist? A review. *Journal of the American Medical Association,* 259:1353-1356.

14. Friedland, G.H., Saltzman, B.R., Rogers, M.F., et al. (1986). Lack of transmission of HTLV-III/LAV infection to household contacts of patients with AIDS or AIDS-related complex with oral candidiasis. *New England Journal of Medicine,* 314:344-349.

15. Denison, S.A., Lemon, S.M., Baker, L.N., et al. (1987). Quantitative analysis of hepatitis B virus DNA in saliva and semen of chronically infected homosexual men. *Journal of Infectious Diseases,* 156:299-306.

16. Cancio-Bello, TP, de Medina, M., Shorey, J., et al. (1982). An institutional outbreak of hepatitis B related to a human biting carrier. *Journal of Infectious Diseases,* 146:652-656.

17. MacQuarrie, M.B., Forghani, B. and Wolochow, D.A. (1974). Hepatitis B transmitted by a human bite. *Journal of the American Medical Association,* 230:723-724.

18. Scott, R.M., Snitbhan, R., Bancroft, W.H., et al. (1980). Experimental

transmission of hepatitis B virus by semen and saliva. *Journal of Infectious Disease,* 142:67-71.

19. Glaser, J.B. and Nadler, J.P. (1985). Hepatitis B virus in a cardiopulmonary resuscitation training course: Risk of transmission from a surface antigen-positive participant. *Archives of Internal Medicine,* 145:1653-1655.

20. Osterholm, M.T., Bravo, E.R., Crosson, J.T., et al. (1979). Lack of transmission of viral hepatitis type B after oral exposure to HBsAg-positive saliva. *British Medical Journal,* 2:1263-1264.

21. Curran, J.W., Jaffe, H.W., Hardy, A.M., et al. (1988). Epidemiology of HIV infection and AIDS in the United States. *Science,* 239:610-616.

22. Jason, J.M., McDougal, J.S., Dixon, G., et al. (1986). HTLV-III/LAV antibody and immuno status of household contacts and sexual partners of persons with hemophilia. *Journal of the American Medical Association,* 255:212-215.

23. Wahn, V., Kramer, H.H., Voit, T., et al. (1986). Horizontal transmission of HIV infection between two siblings (Letter). *Lancet,* 2:694.

24. Salahuddin, S.Z., Groopman, J.E., Markham, P.D., et al. (1984). HTLV-III in symptom-free seronegative persons. *Lancet,* 2:1418-1420.

25. Simmons, B.P. and Wong, E.S. (1982). *Guideline for Prevention of Nosocomial Pneumonia.* Atlanta: US Department of Health and Human Services, Public Health Service, Centers for Disease Control.

26. Klein, R.S., Phelan, J.A., Freeman, K., et al. (1988). Low occupational risk of human immunodeficiency virus infection among dental professionals. *New England Journal of Medicine,* 318:86-90.

27. Garner, J.S. and Favero, M.S. (1985). *Guideline for Handwashing and Hospital Environmental Control, 1985.* Atlanta: US Department of Health and Human Services, Public Health Service, Centers for Disease Control: HHS Publication no. 99-1117.

28. Centers for Disease Control (1988). 1988 Agent summary statement for human immunodeficiency virus and report on laboratory-acquired infection with human immunodeficiency virus. *Morbidity and Mortality Weekly Report,* 37(Suppl no. S4):1S-22S.

Appendix D

Opportunistic Diseases Frequently Associated with AIDS

Protozoal/Parasitic

Pneumocystis carinii pneumonia (PCP) - one of the most frequent causes of death in PWAs. Pneumocystis is ubiquitous and is normally benign in the presence of a healthy immune system. In persons with a compromised immune system Pneumocystis may develop, usually attacking the lungs, causing pneumonia. Pneumocystis is now routinely treated with pentamidine.

Toxoplasma gondii - the host of this protozoa is the cat, and it is found in over 50 percent of the adult population, where it is typically benign. However, in PWAs, it can cause brain abscess, encephalitis and myocarditis. It is a known teratogen if passed to a developing fetus. It can be transmitted by cat handling, contact with cat feces and contact with firewood. Transmission of *Toxoplasma gondii* can be interrupted by vigorous handwashing.

Cryptosporidium difficile - found in the intestines of animals, it lodges in the intestines of humans and can cause profound diarrhea. While seen more frequently in persons with compromised immune systems, it is also prevalent in healthy individuals, as well.

Strongyloidosis - infestation with a genus of roundworms which are typically found in the intestines, and is usually a cause of chronic diarrhea in patients with AIDS. It may also cause pneumonia in these individuals.

Fungal Infections

Cryptococcus neoformans - can be found in a number of body systems resulting in pneumonia, meningitis, lymphadenopathy, endocarditis, nephritis and skin ulcers. Cryptococcus can be transmitted by way of pigeon feces.

*Candidiasis (candida albican/***thrush**) - affects the mucous membranes, skin and internal organs. It is frequently seen in the mouth and esophagus, causing dysphagia. It can also be found in the nailbeds, armpits and anus. Internally, it can be found in the lungs, heart and meninges. In healthy men and women, it is often a common cause of genital infections.

Histoplasma capsulatum (**histoplasmosis**) - found in the lungs. It may cause emaciation, irregular fever, leukopenia and splenomegaly.

Aspergillosis - affects mucous membranes and may be found throughout the body, including the lungs, eyes, nose, ears, liver, kidneys and urethra.

Viral Infections

Cytomegalovirus (CMV) - related to the herpes virus. Affects eyes (causing retinitis), gastrointestinal (GI) tract, CNS and lungs. CMV is characteristically latent for long periods of time. It is present in 50 percent of the general population between the ages of 18 and 25, and in 80 percent of those over the age of 35. CMV produces mild, flu-like symptoms and is usually self-limiting. Severe cases may produce hepatitis, mononucleosis, or pneumonia, even in healthy individuals. It is a teratogen. Transmission is by way of body fluids. Again, handwashing will interrupt transmission.

Herpes simplex virus (HSV I) - commonly causes cold sores and fever blisters, primarily in and around the mouth. Herpes viruses can lie dormant for long periods of time within the relative protection of the CNS where they are protected from the immune system.

Herpes simplex virus II (HSV II) - venereal herpes/genital herpes. Causes painful lesions on genital and anus. Can also be transmitted to face and mouth. In newborns and individuals with impaired immune systems, the disease can be quite severe and frequently causes death.

Herpes varicella-zoster virus (HVZ) - causes chicken pox in children and may reprise as shingles in adults. As shingles, the virus follows nerve trunks and causes extremely painful blisters on the skin. HVZ can cause pneumonia and encephalitis in persons with compromised immune systems. HVZ can be transmitted by contact with blisters and care should be taken to avoid transmission in this manner.

Epstein-Barr Virus (EBV) - this virus typically causes mononucleosis and is spread by kissing. EBV lies dormant in lymph glands and has been associated with some lymphomas.

Bacterial Infections

Mycobacterium avium intracellulare (MAI) - affects lungs, bone, lymph nodes, liver and spleen. MAI can cause extremely high fevers of as high as 106 F.

Nocardiosis - infection by the genus *Nocardia asteroides* typically begins as a pulmonary infection causing a cough with thick sputum. It may also cause extremely high fevers, chills, night sweats, anorexia, malaise, and weight loss. Infection can spread to the brain by way of the circulatory system where abscesses may form, resulting in confusion, disorientation, headache, nausea and seizures. The infection may also cause endocarditis, as well as disorders of the liver, spleen, bones, and subcutaneous tissue.

Shigella flexneri (**shigellosis**) - causes diarrhea and fatal dysentery. Complications of shigellosis may include electrolyte imbalance, metabolic acidosis and shock.

Salmonella enteritidis (salmonellosis) - causes gastroenteritis, diarrhea and bacteremia. It also affects brain and bone tissue.

Neoplasms

Kaposi's sarcoma (KS) - typically seen in older individuals of Mediterranean descent, the lesions are most often found only on the lower extremities. When KS is a manifestation of AIDS, it usually effects primarily gay men, and the lesions, which can be extremely disfiguring, can be found anywhere on the skin. These lesions can also be found to effect numerous internal organs, as well.

Lymphoma - lymphomas can include Hodgkin's disease, non-Hodgkin's lymphoma, and Burkitt's lymphoma.

References

Cahill, K.M. (Ed.) (1983). *The AIDS Epidemic*. New York: St. Martin's Press.

Clayton, L.T. (Ed.) (1985). *Tabers Cyclopedic Medical Dictionary* 15th ed. Philadelphia: F.A. Davis.

Cuff, M. (nd). *Infections frequently associated with AIDS*. New York: Gay Men's Health Crisis.

Rubin, A.M. and West, R.S. (eds.) (1982). *Professional Guide to Diseases*. Springhouse, PA: Intermed Communications.

Appendix E

AIDS Resources

State and Local Organizations

ALABAMA
Alabama Department of Public Health
Division of AIDS Prevention and Control
434 Monroe Street, Room 756
Montgomery, AL 36130-1701
(205) 261-5838

Alabama AIDS Resource Directory
Alabama AIDS Prevention Network
University of South Alabama, Department of Pathology
2451 Filingim Street
Mobile, AL 36617
(205) 471-7322

ALASKA
Alaska Department of Health and Social Services
Division of Public Health
Epidemiology Section
Alaska AIDS Program
3601 C Street, Suite 540
Anchorage, AK
(907) 561-4406

ARIZONA
Arizona Department of Health Services
Division of Disease Prevention
AIDS Section
3008 North 3rd Street, Room 103
Phoenix, AZ 85021
(602) 230-5833

Maricopa County Client Services Directory
Arizona AIDS Project
736 East Flynn Lane
Phoenix, AZ 85014
(602) 277-1929

ARKANSAS
Arkansas Department of Health
Sexually Transmitted Diseases Division
4815 West Markham, Room 455
Little Rock, AR 72205
(501) 661-2133

CALIFORNIA
California Department of Health Services
Office of AIDS
714-744 P Street
Sacramento, CA 94234
(916) 445 0553

Directory of AIDS Services
AIDS Project/Los Angeles
3670 Wilshire Boulevard
Los Angeles, CA 90010
(213) 738-8200

AIDS & ARC: A Guide to Resources in Orange County
AIDS Response Program/AIDS Service Foundation
12832 Garden Grove Boulevard, Suite E
Garden Grove, CA 92643

San Diego County AIDS Directory
San Diego County Regional Task Force on AIDS
c/o Department of Health Services
1700 Pacific Highway
San Diego, CA 92101
(619) 236-2705

AIDS and ARC: A Resource Manual
San Francisco AIDS Foundation
333 Valencia Street
San Francisco, CA 94103
(415) 864-4376

COLORADO
Colorado Department of Health
Sexually Transmitted Diseases/AIDS Control
4210 East 11th Avenue
Denver, CO 80220
(303) 331-8320

CONNECTICUT
AIDS: A Resource Guide for Connecticut
Connecticut Department of Health Services
AIDS Program
150 Washington Street
Hartford, CT 06106
(203) 566-1157

DELAWARE
Delaware Department of Health and Social Services
Division of Public Health
Bureau of Disease Control
AIDS Program Office
3000 Newport Gap Pike, Building G
Wilmington, DE 19808
(302) 995-8422

DISTRICT OF COLUMBIA
District of Columbia Department of Human Services
Commission of Public Health
Office of AIDS Activities
1875 Connecticut Avenue, NW
Washington, DC 20036
(202) 673-6888

FLORIDA
Florida Department of Health and Rehabilitative Services
AIDS Program
1317 Winewood Boulevard, Building 6
Tallahassee, FL 32399-0700
(904) 487-2478

Directory of AIDS Services
Tampa AIDS Network
P.O. Box 1062
Tampa, FL 33601
(813) 221-6420

GEORGIA
Georgia Department of Human Services
Division of Public Health
Community Health Section, AIDS Unit
878 Peachtree St., NE, Room 102
Atlanta, GA 30309
(404) 894-6428

HAWAII
Hawaii Department of Health
AIDS Sexually Transmitted Disease Control Branch
3627 Kilauea Avenue, Suite 304
Honolulu, HI 96816
(808) 735-5303

IDAHO
Idaho Department of Health and Welfare
Bureau of Preventative Medicine
AIDS Drug Reimbursement Program
450 West State Street
Boise, ID 83720
(208) 334-5932

AIDS Resource List
Idaho AIDS Program
450 West State Street
Boise, ID 83720
(208) 334-5937

ILLINOIS
Illinois Department of Public Health
Division of Infectious Diseases
AIDS Activity Section
100 West Randolph Street, Suite 6-600
Chicago, IL 60601
(312) 917-4846

INDIANA
AIDS: Community Resources Directory
Indiana State Board of Health
AIDS Activity Office
1330 West Michigan Street
Indianapolis, IN 46206
(317) 633-0851

IOWA
Iowa Department of Public Health
Division of Disease Prevention
AIDS Program
Lucas State Office Building
Des Moines, IA 50319-0075
(515) 281-4938

KANSAS

Kansas Department of Health and Environment
Division of Health Bureau of Epidemiology
AIDS Bureau Reimbursement Program
Mills Building, Suite 605
109 S.W. 9th
Topeka, KS 66612-1271
(913) 296-5586

KENTUCKY

Kentucky Department of Health Services
Communicable Disease Branch
AIDS Program
275 East Main St., 2nd Floor, East
Frankfort, KY 40621
(502) 564-4804

LOUISIANA

Louisiana Department of Health and Hospitals
Office of Public Health
AIDS Prevention and Surveillance Program
P.O. Box 60630, Room 618
New Orleans, LA 70160
(504) 568-5508

AIDS Referral List
New Orleans Health Department
1300 Perdido St., Room 8E13
New Orleans, LA 70112
(504) 586-4665

MAINE

Maine Department of Human Services
Division of Communicable Disease Control
AIDS Prevention Grant Project
State House Sta.
Augusta, ME 04330
(207) 289-3747

MARYLAND

Maryland Department of Health and Mental Hygiene
Center for AIDS Related Educational Services
201 West Preston St.
Baltimore, MD 21202
(301) 225-6707

MASSACHUSETTS
Massachusetts Department of Public Health
Division of Commonwealth Disease Control
AIDS Program
305 South St.
Jamaica Plain, MA 02130
(617) 522-3700

MICHIGAN
Michigan Department of Public Health
Center for Health Promotion
Special Office on AIDS Prevention
3423 North Logan St.
Lansing, MI 48909
(517) 335-8371

MINNESOTA
Minnesota Department of Health
Division of Disease Prevention and Health Promotion
AIDS Prevention Services Section
717 Delaware Street, SE
Minneapolis, MN 55440
(612) 623-5662

*AIDS Related Resources for Referral in Minnesota**
Minnesota AIDS Project
2025 Nicollet Avenue, South, #200
Minneapolis, MN 55404
(612) 870-7773

MISSISSIPPI
Mississippi Department of Health
AIDS/HIV Prevention Program
2423 North State Street
Jackson, MS 39215-1700
(601) 960-7723

MISSOURI
Missouri Department of Health
Bureau of AIDS Prevention
1730 East Elm
Jefferson City, MO 65102
(314) 751-6438

MONTANA

Montana Department of Health and Environmental Sciences
AIDS/STD Program
1400 Broadway
Cogswell Building
Helena, MT 59620
(406) 444-4740

NEBRASKA

Nebraska Department of Health
AIDS Program
P.O. Box 95007
Lincoln, NE 68509-5007
(402) 471-4091

NEVADA

Nevada AIDS Resource List
Nevada State Health Division AIDS Program
Capitol Complex
Carson City, NV 89710
(702) 885-4800

NEW HAMPSHIRE

AIDS: The Resource Guide for New Hampshire
New Hampshire Department of Health and Welfare
6 Hazen Drive
Concord, NH 03301
(603) 271-4490

NEW JERSEY

New Jersey Department of Health, Prevention, Training and
Education, AIDS Program
CN 363
363 West State Street
Trenton, NJ 08625
(609) 984-6000

NEW MEXICO

New Mexico AIDS Information and Services
New Mexico Health and Environment Department
AIDS Prevention Program
P.O. Box 968
Sante Fe, NM 87504
(505) 827-0090

NEW YORK
New York Department of Health
Office of Public Health, AIDS Institute
Corning Tower, #359
1315 Empire State Plaza
Albany, NY 12237
(518) 473-7238

AIDS Resource Manual
New York State Department of Social Services
Professional Development Program
Rockefeller College, SUNY Albany
Albany, NY 12222
(518) 442-5715

AIDS: A Resource Guide for New York City
New York City Department of Health
Division of Health Promotion
125 Worth Street
New York, NY 10013
(212) 566-7103

NORTH CAROLINA
North Carolina Department of Human Resources
Division of Health Services
P.O. Box 2091
Raleigh, NC 27602-2091
(919) 733-3419

NORTH DAKOTA
North Dakota Department of Health
Division of Disease Control
AIDS Program
600 East Boulevard
Bismarck, ND 58505-0200
(701) 224-2378

OHIO
Ohio Department of Health
Epidemiology Division
246 North High Street
Columbus, OH 43266-0588
(614) 466-5480

AIDS Resource Directory
Northeast Ohio Task Force on AIDS
177 South Broadway
Akron, OH 44308
(216) 375-2960

OKLAHOMA
Oklahoma Department of Health
AIDS Division
100 NE 10th
Oklahoma City, OK 73152
(405) 271-4636

Resource Guide for Patients with AIDS/ARC
Tulsa AIDS Task Force/Oklahoma Department of Health
P.O. Box 4330
Tulsa, OK 74159

OREGON
Oregon Department of Human Resources
Health Division, AIDS Program
1400 NE 5th Avenue
Portland, OR 97201
(503) 229-5792

PENNSYLVANIA
Pennsylvania Department of Health
AIDS Program
P.O. Box 90, Room 813
Harrisburg, PA 17108
(717) 783-0479

RHODE ISLAND
Rhode Island Department of Health
AIDS Program
75 Davis Street
Providence, RI 02908
(401) 277-2362

SOUTH CAROLINA
South Carolina Department of Health & Environmental Control
Bureau of Preventative Health Services
AIDS Prevention Project
2600 Bull Street
Columbia, SC 29201
(803) 734-5482

SOUTH DAKOTA
AIDS Resource List
South Dakota Department of Health
Communicable Disease Program
523 East Capitol
Pierre, SD 57501
(605) 773-3364

TENNESSEE
AIDS: Information, Education, Testing, Counseling
Tennessee Department of Health and Environment
Tennessee Hospital Association
100 Ninth Avenue, North
Nashville, TN 37219
(615) 741-7387

TEXAS
Texas Department of Health
Bureau of AIDS and Sexually Transmitted Disease Control
AIDS Division
1100 West 49th Street
Austin, TX 78756
(512) 458-7207

UTAH
Utah AIDS Resource Directory
Utah Department of Health
Division of Community Health Services
P.O. Box 16660
Salt Lake City, UT 84116
(801) 538-6191

VERMONT
Vermont Department of Health
Division of Epidemiology AIDS Program
60 Main Street
Burlington, VT 05402
(802) 863-7200

VIRGINIA
Virginia Department of Health
Division of Communicable Disease Control
Sexually Transmitted Disease/AIDS Control
109 Governor Street
Richmond, VA 23219
(804) 786-6267

WASHINGTON
Washington Department of Health
Office on HIV/AIDS
Airdustrial Park, Building 9
Mail Stop LJ-17
Olympia, WA 98504
(206) 586-0426

WEST VIRGINIA
West Virginia Department of Health
Office of Epidemiology and Health Promotion Division of
Surveillance and Disease Control AIDS Prevention Program
151 11th Avenue
South Charleston, WV 25305
(304) 348-2950

WISCONSIN
Wisconsin AIDS Update
Wisconsin Department of Health and Social Services
Division of Health
1 West Wilson Street
Madison, WI 53701
(608) 266-9853

WYOMING
AIDS Resource Manual
Wyoming Division of Health and Medical Services
AIDS Risk Reduction Program
Hathaway Building
Cheyenne, WY 82002
(307) 777-7953

United States Territories

American Samoa Department of Health Services
AIDS Drug Reimbursement Program
LBJ Tropical Medical Center
Pago Pago, AS 96799
(684) 633-5743

Guam Department of Public Health and Social Services
AIDS Drug Reimbursement Program
P.O. Box 2816
Agana, GU 96910
(671) 734-2947

Puerto Rico Department of Health
Sexually Transmitted Disease Program
Call Box STD
San Juan, PR 00922
(809) 754-8118

Virgin Islands Department of Health
Community Health Services
AIDS Drug Reimbursement Program
P.O. Box 1026
St. Croix, VI 00820
(809) 776-8311

Private and Community Based AIDS Organizations

Academy for Educational Development
AIDSCOM
1255 23rd Street, Suite 400
Washington, DC 20037
(202) 862-1900

ADAPT—Association for Drug Abuse and Treatment
88 Bergen Street
Brooklyn, NY 11201
(718) 834-9585

AID Atlanta
1132 West Peachtree Street, NW
Atlanta, GA 30309
(404) 872-0600

AIDS Action Committee
131 Clarendon Street, 5th Floor
Boston, MA 02116
(617) 437-6200

AIDS Action Committee
2033 M Street, NW, 8th Floor
Washington, DC 20036
(202) 547-3101

AIDS Foundation of Houston
3927 Essex Lane
Houston, TX 77027
(713) 623-6796

AIDS Project/Los Angeles
3670 Wilshire Boulevard, Suite 300
Los Angeles, CA 90010
(213) 738-8200

American National Red Cross
1730 D Street, NW
Washington, DC 20006
(202) 639-3004

American Psychological Association
AIDS Community Training Project
1200 17th Street, NW
Washington, DC 20036
(202) 955-7740

American Public Health Association
1015 15th Street, NW
Washington, DC 20005
(202) 789-5600

BEBASHI—Blacks Educating Blacks About Sexual Health Issues
1528 Walnut Street, Suite 1414
Philadelphia, PA 19102
(215) 546-4140

Cascade AIDS Project
408 SW 2nd, Suite 412
Portland, OR 97204
(503) 223-5907

Colorado AIDS Project
P.O. Box 18529
Denver, CO 80218
(303) 837-0166

Gay Men's Health Crisis
129 West 20th Street
New York, NY 10010
(212) 807-6655

HERO—Health Education and Resource Organization
101 West Read Street, Suite 800
Baltimore, MD 21201
(301) 685-1180

Health Issues Task Force
3130 Mayfield Road, #306
Cleveland Heights, OH 44118
(216) 371-5111

Hispanic AIDS Forum
140 22nd Street
New York, NY 10010
(212) 966-6662

Intergovernmental Health Policy Project
2100 Pennsylvania Avenue, NW
Washington, DC 20037
(202) 872-1445

Lambda Legal Defense and Education Fund
666 Broadway, 12th Floor
New York, NY 10012
(212) 995-8585

Milwaukee AIDS Project
P.O. Box 92505
Milwaukee, WI 53202
(414) 273-AIDS

Minnesota AIDS Project
2025 Nicollet South, Suite 200
Minneapolis, MN 55403
(612) 870-7773

National AIDS Hotline
1-800-342-AIDS

National AIDS Network
2033 M Street, NW, Suite 800
Washington, DC 20036
(202) 293-2437

National Association of People with AIDS
2025 I Street, NW, Suite 415
Washington, DC 20006
(202) 429-2856

National Coalition of Black Lesbians and Gays
19641 West Seven Mile Road
Detroit, MI 48219
(313) 897-9079

National Coalition of Gay STD Services
P.O. Box 239
Milwaukee, WI 53201
(414) 277-7671

National Coalition of Hispanic Health and Human Service Organizations
1030 15th Street, NW, Suite 1053
Washington, DC 20005
(202) 371-2100

National Community Research Initiative
P.O. Box 29058
Washington, DC 20017-0058
(202) 529-9187

National Council of La Raza
20 F Street, NW, 2nd Floor
Washington, DC 20001
(202) 628-9600

National Gay and Lesbian Task Force
1517 U Street, NW
Washington, DC 20009
(202) 332-6483

National Hemophilia Foundation
SoHo Building
110 Greene Street, Room 406
New York, NY 10012
(212) 219-8180

National Institutes of Health
Toll-free hotline for
federal government clinical trial information
1-800-TRIALS-A

National Jewish AIDS Project
1082 Columbia Road, Suite 32
Washington, DC 20009
(202) 387-3097

National Lawyers Guild AIDS Project
211 Gough Street, Suite 311
San Francisco, CA 94102
(415) 861-8884

National Leadership Coalition on AIDS
1150 15th Street, NW, Suite 202
Washington, DC 20036
(202) 429-0930

National Lesbian and Gay Health Foundation
P.O. Box 65472
Washington, DC 20035
(202) 797-3708

National Minority AIDS Council
714 G Street, SE
Washington, DC 20003
(202) 544-1076

Northwest AIDS Foundation
818 East Pike
Seattle, WA 98122
(206) 329-6923

PWA Coalition
31 West 26th Street
New York, NY 10010
Hotline (staffed by PWA/ARCs)
10:00 am–8:00 on EST, Mon-Thurs
10:00 am–6:00 pm Friday
(212) 532-0568
1-800-828-3280

San Francisco AIDS Foundation
25 Van Ness Avenue, Suite 660
San Francisco, CA 94103
(415) 864-5855

U.S. Conference of Mayors
AIDS Program
1620 Eye Street, NW
Washington, DC 20001
(202) 293-7330

Whitman Walker Clinic AIDS Program
1407 S Street, NW
Washington, DC 20009
(202) 797-3540

AIDS Publications

AIDS Alert
American Health Consultants
67 Peachtree Park Drive, NE
Atlanta, GA 30309
(404) 351-4523

AIDS & Public Policy Journal
University Publishing Group
107 East Church Street
Frederick, MD 21701
(800) 654-8188

AIDS Clinical Digest
American Health Consultants
67 Peachtree Park Drive, NE
Atlanta, GA 30309
(404) 351-4523

AIDS Forum
P.O. Box 6400
Scottsdale, AZ
(602) 994-0182

AIDS Information Exchange
U.S. Conference of Mayors
1620 Eye Street, NW
Washington, DC 20006
(202) 293-7330

AIDS Literature and News Review
University Publishing Group
107 East Church Street
Frederick, MD 21701
(800) 654-8188

AIDS Monthly Surveillance Report
Centers for Disease Control
1600 Clifton Road
Atlanta, GA 30333

AIDS Patient Care
Mary Ann Liebert Publishers
1651 Third Avenue
New York, NY 10128
(212) 289-2300

AIDS Policy and Law
Bureau of National Affairs
2445 M Street, NW, Suite 275
Washington DC 20037
(202) 452-7889

AIDS Record
BioData Publishers
1347 30th Street, NW
Washington, DC 20007
(202) 393-2437

AIDS Treatment Data Network
(Treatment information in English
and Spanish)
259 W 30th Street
New York, NY 10011
(212) 268-4196

AIDS Treatment News
P.O. Box 411256
San Francisco, CA 94141
(415) 255-0588

*AMFAR Experimental Treatment
Directory*
1515 Broadway, Suite 3601
New York, NY 10036
(212) 719-0033

Body Positive, The
(A magazine for sero-positives)
2095 Broadway, Suite 306
New York, NY 10023
(212) 721-1346

*Bulletin of Experimental Treatments for
AIDS (BETA)*
San Francisco AIDS Foundation
P.O. Box 6182
San Francisco, CA 94101
(415) 863-AIDS

COSSMHO AIDS Update
1030 15th Street, NW
85261 Suite 1053
Washington, DC 20005
(202) 371-2100

FOCUS
AIDS Health Project
333 Valencia Street, 4th Floor
San Francisco, CA 94103

Journal of Acquired Immune Deficiency Syndrome
Raven Press
1185 Avenue of the Americas
New York, NY 10036

Morbidity and Mortality Weekly Reports (MMWR)
Centers for Disease Control
1600 Clifton Road
Atlanta, GA 30333

Multicultural Inquiry and Research on AIDS (MIRA)
6025 Third Street
San Francisco, CA 94214
(415) 822-4030

Multi-Cultural NOTES
National AIDS Network
2033 M Street, NW, Suite 800
Washington, DC 20036
(202) 293-2437

NAN Monitor
National AIDS Network
2033 M Street, NW, Suite 800
Washington, DC 20036
(202) 293-2437

Notes From the Underground
PWA Health Group Newsletter
150 W 26th Street
New York, NY 10010
(212) 255-0520

PI Perspective and *Fact Sheets*
Project Inform
347 Delores Street, Suite 301
San Francisco, CA 94110
1-800-822-7422

PWA Coalition Newsline
PWA Coalition
263 West 19th Street, #125
New York, NY 10011
(212) 627-1810

SIDAhora
(Bilingual publication)
PWA Coalition
31 W 26th Street
New York, NY 10010

Treatment Update
Treatment Information Exchange,
AIDS Action Now!
517 College Steet, Suite 324
Toronto, Ontario M6G 1A8
CANADA
(416) 944-1916

Vancouver PWA Society Newsletter
1447 Hornby Street
Vancouver, British Columbia
V6Z 1W8
CANADA
(604) 683-3381

Answers to AIDS Self-Knowledge Test

1.	False	11.	True
2.	True	12.	True
3.	False	13.	False
4.	False	14.	True
5.	True	15.	True
6.	False	16.	True
7.	True	17.	True
8.	False	18.	True
9.	False	19.	False
10.	False	20.	False

Glossary of Abbreviations and Acronyms

AA	after AIDS.
ACIP	Immunization Practices Advisory Committee.
ADL	activities of daily living.
ADS	AIDS dementia complex.
AFB	acid fast bacillus.
AFO	ankle-foot orthosis.
AIDS	acquired immunodeficiency syndrome.
AMA	American Medical Association.
AMSAODD	American Medical Society on Alcoholism and Other Drug Dependence.
AOTA	American Occupational Therapy Association.
ARC	AIDS-related complex.
AZT	azidothymidine.
BA	before AIDS.
BEA	bacillary epithelial angiomatosis.
CDC	Centers for Disease Control.
COBRA	Consolidated Omnibus Budget Reconciliation Act.
CMV	cytomegalovirus.
CRI	Community Research Institute.
CSF	cerebrospinal fluid.
CSTE	Council of State and Territorial Epidemiologists.
CT	computed tomography.
CVA	cardiovascular accident.
DDI	dideoxyinosine.
DHPG	dihydroxypropoxymethyl guanine (ganciclovir).
DNA	deoxyribonucleic acid.
EIA	enzyme immunoassay.

ELISA	enzyme-linked immunosorbent assay.
EPA	Environmental Protection Agency.
FDA	Food and Drug Administration.
GI	gastrointestinal.
GP	glycoprotein.
GRIDS	gay-related immune deficiency syndrome.
GST	general systems theory.
GW	George Washington University.
HBsAG	hepatitis B surface antigen.
HBV	hepatitis B virus.
HHS	Health and Human Services.
HIV	human immunodeficiency virus.
HSV	herpes simplex virus.
HTLV-II	human T-lymphotropic virus isolate III.
HVZ	herpes varicella zoster virus.
IC	infection control.
IDDM	insulin dependent diabetes mellitus.
IV	intravenous.
IVDA	intravenous drug abuser.
IVDU	intravenous drug user.
KS	Kaposi's sarcoma.
LAV	lymphadenopathy-associated virus.
LIP	lymphoid interstitial pneumonia.
LIP/PLH	lymphoid interstitial pneumonia and/or pulmonary lymphoid hyperplasia (complex).
LUE	left upper extremity.
MAI	*Mycobacterium avium intracellulare.*
MIB	Medical Information Bureau.
MRI	magnetic resonance imaging.
NDT	neurodevelopmental therapy.
OSHA	Occupational Safety and Health Administration.
OT	occupational therapy.
PCA	personal care aide.
PCP	*Pneumocystis carinii* pneumonia.
PCR	polymerized chain reaction.
PGL	persistent generalized lymphadenopathy.
PHS	Public Health Service.
PLH	pulmonary lymphoid hyperplasia.

PNF	proprioceptive neuromuscular facilitation.
PRE	progressive resistive exercises.
PWA	person with AIDS.
PWARC	person with AIDS-related complex.
RNA	ribonucleic aid.
RUE	right upper extremity.
SSDI	Social Security Disability Income.
SSI	Supplemental Social Security.
STD	sexually transmitted disease.
SUDS	single-use diagnostic system.
TB	tuberculosis.
TENS	transcutaneous nerve stimulators.
VD	venereal disease.
VD/STD	venereal disease/sexually transmitted disease.
VZV	variella zoster virus.

Glossary

Acquired Immune Deficiency Syndrome (AIDS) — the final stage of HIV infection. AIDS is manifested by a positive ELISA and/or Western blot test, a T-cell count of less than 400 cells/mm^3, and the presence of certain opportunistic infections, specifically, *Pneumocystis carinii* pneumonia (PCP), and Kaposi's sarcoma. In 1987 the Centers for Disease Control (CDC) expanded the definition to include HIV encephalopathy and HIV wasting syndrome.

Acyclovir — a drug used to control recurrent episodes of the herpes simplex virus (HSV). It is not a cure for HSV.

AIDS Related Complex (ARC) — an advanced stage of HIV infection. ARC is typically manifested by chronic fever, chronic diarrhea and soaking night sweats.

Azidothymidine (AZT) — one of two federally approved drugs used to treat HIV disease. AZT disrupts the replication of HIV by interrupting the viral DNA chain and thus retards the progression of the disease. Side effects of AZT may include nausea, abdominal cramps, headaches and anemia. AZT is produced by Burroughs-Wellcome and is sold under the trade name of Zidovudine.

Body Fluids — fluids that have been recognized by the CDC as directly linked to the transmission of HIV and/or HBV and/or to which universal precautions apply: blood, semen, blood products, vaginal secretions, cerebrospinal fluid, synovial fluid, pleural fluid, peritoneal fluid, pericardial fluid, amniotic fluid, and concentrated HIV or HBV viruses.

CD-4 — a molecule contained on the cell membrane of certain cells, including T-4 helper lymphocytes and glial cells in the central nervous system, for which HIV appears to have an affinity. CD-4 is considered to be a possible treatment for HIV infection. Theoretically, by administering genetically engineered CD-4 to an infected individual, HIV will be attracted to, and bind with it, thus preventing viral invasion of potential host cells and replication.

Compound Q (GLQ-223) — a highly purified protein from the Chinese cucumber *Trichosanthes kirilowii* which is being considered as a possible treatment for HIV infection. Compound Q has been found to inhibit HIV replication in vitro by selectively destroying HIV-infected macrophages and T cells.

Dideooxyinosine (DDI) — the second of two federally approved drugs used to treat HIV disease. Licensed in September 1989, DDI is chemically related to, but less effective than, AZT. However, it is also less toxic and has fewer side effects. DDI is produced by Bristol-Myers.

Enzyme-Linked Immunoabsorbant Assay (ELISA) — a serologic test used to demonstrate the presence of HIV antibodies. The ELISA does not detect the virus itself. It is a relatively inexpensive and quick test. A positive ELISA is verified by a Western blot test.

Fluconazole — a drug approved by the Food and Drug Administration in early 1990 for treatment of cryptococcal meningitis and candiasis.

Health-Care Worker — an employee of a health care facility including, but not limited to, nurses, physicians, dentists and other dental workers, optometrists, podiatrists, chiropractors, laboratory and blood bank technologists and technicians, research laboratory scientists, phlebotomists, dialysis personnel, paramedics, emergency medical technicians, medical examiners, morticians, housekeepers, laundry workers and others whose work may involve direct contact with body fluids from living individuals or corpses. (From OSHA CPL 2-2.44A.)

HIV Disease — any stage of disease that is caused by infection with the human immunodeficiency virus (HIV). These stages include HIV-positive, asymptomatic, persistent generalized lymphadenopathy (PGL), AIDS-related complex (ARC), and acquired immune deficiency syndrome (AIDS).

HIV AG-1 — a serologic test, approved by the FDA in 1989, which tests for HIV protein levels in the blood.

HIV-Positive, asymptomatic — a term used to describe an individual who demonstrates the presence of HIV antibodies by way of serologic tests, but who appears healthy and shows no overt symptoms of disease. Persons who are HIV-positive, asymptomatic may or may not progress to further stages of HIV disease, although many frequently do.

Human Immunodeficiency Virus (HIV) — a virus belonging to the family of retroviruses which invades and proliferates within cells associated with the immune system. HIV is attracted to cells containing CD-4 molecules on their protein coats and thus gains entry into the cell. Once inside, HIV may lie dormant for an extended period of time until it is triggered to replicate. The exact triggering mechanism is not fully understood. HIV replicates by transforming its RNA genetic code into that of the host cell's DNA genetic code. It then utilizes the hosts organelles as its own, exhausting and eventually destroying the host. When the host cell dies, it explodes and releases many new viruses which seek new hosts. As the number of host cells are depleted, the immune system is compromised and the body is made vulnerable to a myriad of opportunistic infections which are normally benign within an intact immune system. HIV is extremely fragile and cannot survive when denied access to a host cell. HIV was originally designated as both human T-lymphotrophic virus, isolate III (HTLV-III), and lymphadenopathy-associated virus (LAV).

Human T-lymphotrophic virus, isolate III (HTLV-III) — a term that ascribed to what is now known as the human immunodeficiency virus (HIV). HTLV-III was discovered by Dr. Robert Gallo in 1984, who determined that it was similar to other (retro)viruses, HTLV-I and HTLV-II, which are associated with certain leukemias in humans. The designation of HTLV-III was dropped in 1987 in favor of HIV.

Ideographic — relating to the characteristics of an individual.

Infection Control (IC) Program — an IC program is the establishment's oral or written policy and implementation of procedures relating to the control of infectious disease hazards where employees may be directly exposed to direct contact with body fluids. (From OSHA CPL 2-2.44A.)

Lymphadenopathy-Associated Virus (LAV) — the name ascribed to what is now known as the human immunodeficiency virus (HIV). LAV was discovered in Paris by Dr. Luc Montagnier in 1984—at approximately the same time as Gallo's discovery of HTLV-III. The designation of LAV was also dropped in 1987 in favor of HIV.

Nomothetic — a system of laws that govern (the ultimate living situation, the family or subculture of the patient).

Opportunistic Disease/infection — any disease/infection which proliferates in the absence of a properly functioning immune system. Many of the causal agents are normally present in the body and/or environment, but are governed by the immune system and, therefore, remain benign. Refer to Appendix D for the most common opportunistic infections associated with AIDS.

Pentamadine — a drug which is used to treat *Pneumocystis carinii* pneumonia (PCP), an opportunistic infection which frequently causes death in persons with AIDS (PWAs) Pentamadine is usually administered in aerosol form, but it can also be administered intravenously.

Persons with AIDS (PWAs) — those individuals who have been diagnosed with AIDS, the most advanced stage of HIV disease.

Persons with AIDS-Related Complex (PWARCs) — those individuals who have been diagnosed with AIDS-related complex (ARC), a precursor of AIDS.

Polymerized Chain Reaction (PCR) — a test used in infants of HIV-infected mothers to determine if the HIV DNA is an inherent part of the child's cell or if it is part of the mother's antibodies to the virus. This is in contrast to the ELISA/Western blot tests, which detect only HIV antibodies.

Retrovir — a trade name for azidothymidine (AZT). Retrovir is now more commonly referred to as Zidovudine.

Retrovirus — any one of a family of viruses that is able to transform its RNA genetic code, via reverse transcriptase, into the DNA genetic code of the host cell, thus allowing it to reproduce. Retroviruses include HTLV-I, HTLV-II, and HIV.

Reverse transcriptase — an enzyme that allows HIV to transform its RNA genetic code into the DNA genetic code of its host cell, to reproduce.

Single-Use Diagnostic System (SUDS) — a new serologic test for HIV antibodies which was approved by the FDA in late 1989. SUDS can be administered, and the results known in less than 30 minutes. Trials with SUDS have demonstrated a 99.8 percent accuracy rate.

Universal Precautions — recommended by the CDC to treat the blood and body fluids of *all* patients as potentially infectious with HIV, HBV, or other blood-borne pathogens, since all potential carriers cannot be readily identified. These precautions include proper barrier protection, handwashing, and disposal contaminated materials and sharp instruments that may have been infected. Universal precautions are intended to prevent health-care workers from parenteral, mucous membrane, and non-intact skin exposures to blood-borne pathogens. Refer to Appendices A and B for details.

Western Blot Test — a highly sensitive and relatively expensive serologic assay which tests for the presence of HIV antibodies. The Western blot takes longer to glean results and is used to confirm a positive ELISA result.

Zidovudine — The trade name for azidothymidine (AZT).

References

Cahill, K.M. (Ed.) (1983). *The AIDS Epidemic*. New York: St. Martin's Press.

Centers for Disease Control (1988). Update: Universal precautions for prevention of transmission of human immunodeficiency virus, hepatitis B virus, and other blood-borne pathogens in health-care settings. *Morbidity and Mortality Weekly Report*, 37(24):377-387.

Clement, M. (1989). Your patients may ask. *AIDS Clinical Care*, 1(3):17-27.

Cuff, M. (nd). *Infections Frequently Associated with AIDS*. New York: Gay Men's Health Crisis.

Office of Health Compliance Assistance (OSHA) (1988). OSHA Instruction CPL 2-2.44A.

Taber, C.W. (1988). *Taber's Cyclopedia Medical Dictionary*, 15th ed. Philadelphia: F.A. Davis

Index